# How to Present Negative Medical News in a Positive Light

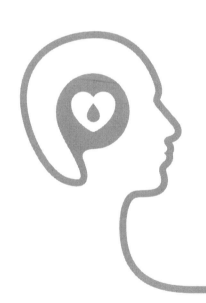

A Prescription
for Health Care
Providers

by Michael J. Cavallaro

# How to Present Negative Medical News in a Positive Light: A Prescription for Health Care Providers

Copyright © 2017 Atlantic Publishing Group, Inc.
1405 SW 6th Avenue • Ocala, Florida 34471 • Phone 800-814-1132 • Fax 352-622-1875
Website: www.atlantic-pub.com • Email: sales@atlantic-pub.com
SAN Number: 268-1250

Library of Congress Cataloging-in-Publication Data

Cavallaro, Michael J., author.
   How to present negative medical news in a positive light : a prescription for health care providers / by Michael J. Cavallaro.
   p. ; cm.
   Includes bibliographical references.
   ISBN-13: 978-1-60138-585-7 (alk. paper)
   ISBN-10: 1-60138-585-4 (alk. paper)
   I. Title.
   [DNLM: 1.  Physician-Patient Relations. 2.  Truth Disclosure. 3.  Communication.  W 62]
   R118
   610.69'6--dc23
                          2013045473

Printed in the United States

PROJECT MANAGER: Rebekah Sack • rsack@atlantic-pub.com
INTERIOR LAYOUT AND JACKET DESIGN: Antoinette D'Amore • addesign@videotron.ca

Printed on Recycled Paper

# Reduce. Reuse.
# RECYCLE.

A decade ago, Atlantic Publishing signed the Green Press Initiative. These guidelines promote environmentally friendly practices, such as using recycled stock and vegetable-based inks, avoiding waste, choosing energy-efficient resources, and promoting a no-pulping policy. We now use 100-percent recycled stock on all our books. The results: in one year, switching to post-consumer recycled stock saved 24 mature trees, 5,000 gallons of water, the equivalent of the total energy used for one home in a year, and the equivalent of the greenhouse gases from one car driven for a year.

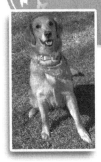 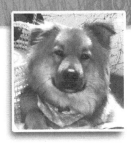 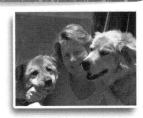

Over the years, we have adopted a number of dogs from rescues and shelters. First there was Bear and after he passed, Ginger and Scout. Now, we have Kira, another rescue. They have brought immense joy and love not just into our lives, but into the lives of all who met them.

We want you to know a portion of the profits of this book will be donated in Bear, Ginger and Scout's memory to local animal shelters, parks, conservation organizations, and other individuals and nonprofit organizations in need of assistance.

**– Douglas & Sherri Brown,**
*President & Vice-President of Atlantic Publishing*

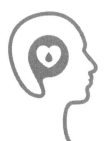

# Dedication

*This book is dedicated to Ella*
*…my companion on the road less travelled.*

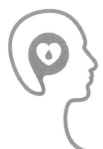

# Disclaimer

*The material in this book is provided for informational purposes and as a general guide to presenting negative medical news to patients and their families. Basic definitions of laws are provided according to the status of the laws at the time of printing; be sure to check for a change or update in laws. This book should not substitute professional and legal counsel for the development of your business.*

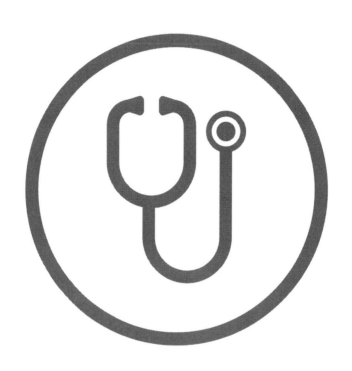

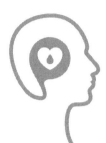# Table of Contents

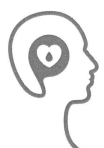

# Introduction

Breaking bad news to patients is a difficult and common part of being a health care provider. While performing this task is common, most physicians, clinicians, oncologists, nurses and other health care practitioners receive almost no training in how to lessen the emotional impact of potentially life-altering news. Worse, the lack of training means most medical providers never see how these applications help the medical practitioner accomplish key goals in managed care. Consider the following quote by Hugh Laurie, who plays the cantankerous Dr. Gregory House on the popular medical drama, *House, M.D.*: "Treating illnesses is why we became doctors. Treating patients is what makes most doctors miserable."

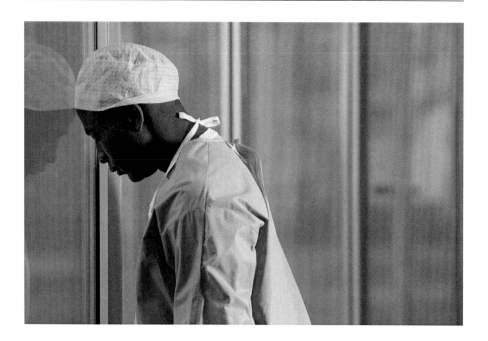

Not to be confused as someone with any bedside manner, it is no surprise that House always finds himself at odds with patients, coworkers, the Hippocratic oath, and the law. Nevertheless, his insights into life are brilliant, and, if his words ring true in your medical experience, this book can help you overcome the typical pitfalls associated with breaking bad news. Learning to apply the methods covered in this book can enhance patient understanding, strengthen patient cooperation, increase patient satisfaction, reduce the time spent dealing with individual cases, and even minimize the possibility of litigation. The topics covered in the first half of this book include the effects of bad news on patients and doctors, strategies for conducting patient interviews, responding to patients, discussing prognosis, and supporting patient decision-making. The topics discussed in the second half of this book include dealing with conflicts, communicating with a patient's family and dealing with interfamilial barriers, ethical issues in communication, communication in palliative and hospice transition, and how to handle postmortem discussions.

Some guidelines discussed in this book apply toward the general practice of breaking bad news in almost any medical situation. Some apply for specific situations, such as breaking news to a patient that an error has occurred in diagnosis, or having to tell a patient that treatments are not working. Additionally, traditional ways in which medical institutions require clinicians to handle their patient relationships today have changed. While the Hippocratic oath written by Hippocrates in late fifth century B.C. is still a covenant sworn by health care practitioners today, the oath was significantly modified in 1948 by the World Medical Association and several times since.

However, no matter how much research in communication and approach has evolved over time, some of the most enduring critiques and grievances expressed about doctors today include the perception that they do not listen to the patient, do not seem to care about the patient, and never admit their errors. Moreover, public opinion confirms the perception that doctors do not take the time to reinforce patient understanding of the illness and management plan. Surprisingly, few doctors consider communication skills important and many don't receive any training for it, yet in most cases, how they handle communication can be to the detriment or benefit of the entire private practice or public institution.

The history of modern communication in health care began in the 1920s with a rhetorical phase of research that did not have a direct impact on the curriculum of medical students. It was not until 1969, when William Morgan and George Engel wrote *The Clinical Approach to the Patient*, that researchers recommended these skills for mandatory assimilation into student curriculums. It was around the same time that Barbara M. Korsch pioneered the first interviews in pediatrics and discovered significant gaps in doctor-patient communication. In the 1970s, Deborah Roter developed the Roter Interaction Analysis System (RIAS), which served as one of the first applications into evaluating verbal interactions between patients and doctors during medical interviews. During the 1980s, Peter Maguire demonstrated proof that early teaching of communication skills to medical students resulted in enduring behaviors that generalized in their careers over time.

Through gradual research and application, doctor-patient relationships eventually shifted from the paternalistic approach of having the doctor make all decisions, to the patient-centered, mutual cooperation approaches of today. Yet, despite these social expectations of modern medicine, a 2009 Gallup poll showed that 30 percent of Americans surveyed believed that the national health care industry offers less-than-good quality of care for its citizens. Clear communication from physicians to patients has become an expectation that our society demands, but one it feels doctors rarely observe. From a clinician, physician, or oncologist perspective, communication skills benefit physicians in meeting key objectives along the illness trajectory. They include helping the patient accept their diagnosis, facilitating an understanding and selection of treatment options according to their health care preferences, creating consideration for medical trials, keeping them as active participants in end-of-life care, and facilitating a dignified death. From a patient perspective, the benefit to having doctors who demonstrate superior communication skills include a greater sense of emotional support through a terrifying ordeal, greater trust in the caregivers, and reduced conflict.

Throughout this book, you will encounter different types of medical conversations that will require sensitive oratory. To address each of these different types of medical conversations, we offer guidelines, or road maps, to maximize your time with the patient, build rapport, turn pessimism into optimism, minimize conflict, reach clinical objectives, and facilitate shared decision-making in accordance with today's patient-centered industry. Additionally, the information contained in this book also will include case studies at the end of each chapter. Each case study is an interview with a professional in the field of medicine, with real accounts of how they communicated bad news to patients. Their insight will help clarify how the topics in each chapter apply in real life or how to handle patient interviews differently under the strategies outlined in this book. Use the information structured in this book by referring to the tables and process tasks for the topical subjects covered in each chapter and in the appendices. We hope you are excited about the possibilities of improving your communication skills with patients. Your patients will thank you for it.

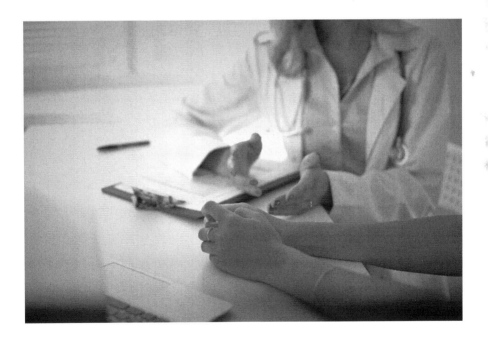

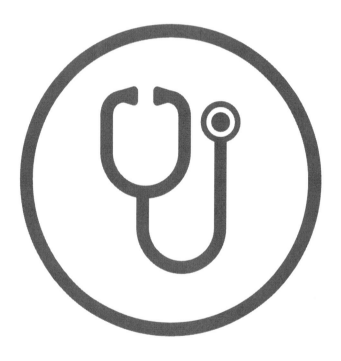

# Chapter 1

# Dynamics of the Doctor/Patient Relationship

he nature of bad news is such that people almost never see it coming. While contingency plans may account for unforeseen situations, life at some point will intervene in a way that defies even careful planning. What we know about life is that everyone makes plans. If you are reading this book, it means you are making specific plans for your professional life, and though considered separate, the plans for your professional life intersect at some point with the plans in your personal life. For example, perhaps you already have met with a financial adviser who has you thinking about a number of important questions about your retirement plans. How much money should you save? Where can you afford to live on the income generated from your work? How do you plan to stay busy when work ends? Do you plan to vacation in the places you did not have time to visit while you worked? Imagine these plans, and then imagine someone delivering news that radically alters your expectations and how you view the future. If you are able to imagine that, you have begun to empathize with patients who hear this on a daily basis. In life, we are amidst death. This is the knowledge people carry with them — that every day, peoples' plans for life are ending and that someday, with absolute certainty, so will ours. This is the primal fear behind any form of bad news, buried deep in the unconscious but always active. It is why the dynamics of the doctor-patient relationship can be so volatile during the initial disclosure of negative medical news. To understand what constitutes bad news, we must first understand its impact. However, we cannot judge its impact unless we understand what patients already know and expect about their life and/or plans.

# Patients: Emotional and Psychological Factors

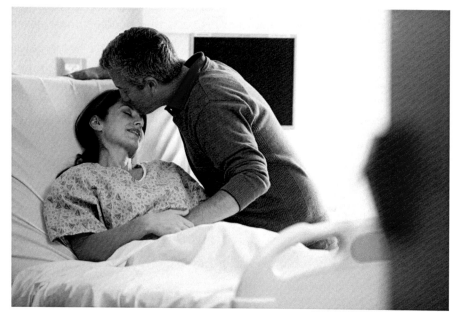

The emotional and psychological factors regulating the effects of receiving bad news may vary from patient to patient. When bad news alters a person's outlook for the future, they may fear that any potential threat to their health status will diminish their freedom or opportunities in life. Because an illness can feature many different symptoms, people experience a multitude of fears and concerns, sometimes grounded in a lack of understanding about the illness, and sometimes grounded in the patient's expectations, ambitions, hopes and beliefs about life. In the case of the former, the doctor's role is to help the patient achieve an understanding about what he or she is facing and what it will mean for their future. In the case of the latter, the doctor's role is to address the emotional and psychological factors affecting the patient by examining reactions to bad news and assessing what the patient specifically needs in order to adjust to the new reality.

While many doctors may view minor, non-fatal diseases and disorders lightly, patients may have a different mindset. The only way to assess the patient's mindset is to examine how the illness relates in context to the individual's life. For example, while a doctor may view a teen diagnosed with genital herpes neutrally because it is non-fatal, common, and treatable, a teen hearing this diagnosis may experience fear due to a lack of medical knowledge or shame for the actions that contributed to the contraction of the disorder. As another example, a bone disorder like osteochondrosis might have a more devastating emotional or psychological impact on a professional runner than someone who works behind a computer, for the obvious reason: a serious bone disorder could alter or destroy a professional runner's livelihood. Therefore, gathering information about a person's entire history before giving bad news enables the doctor to understand its probable effect. As we will explore in Chapter 5, a patient's entire history not only includes an assessment of their medical history, but also their psychohistory.

In cases of serious illness where death is a possible result, the emotional and psychological effect plays straight into the unconscious but always active primal fear previously mentioned. The fear of death triggers strong emotional responses, which, as we will explore in the next few pages, can be a subset of other emotions and are important to identify. When it comes to serious illness, fear is the most common emotion. The different types of patient fears about serious illness include:

- The fear of physical illness
- The fear of its psychological effects
- The fear of death
- The fears associated with treatment
- The fears associated with family and friends
- The fears associated with their social and professional life

The fear of physical illness arises from concerns about physical symptoms. Physical symptoms may vary from minor (e.g. nausea) to severe (e.g. paralysis). However, what the patient considers minor or severe is proportionate to the emotional impact and to its context in their life. The fear of psychological effects relate to one's fear of not being mentally strong enough to cope with the illness, the strain of imagining worst-case scenarios down the line, or the fear of the physical aspect of the illness severely impairing their mental functions (a common psychological fear of patients diagnosed with Alzheimer's).

The fear of death relates to the patient's views on spirituality and existential concerns. The fear of treatments relate to anxieties surrounding the side effects incurred by treatments. Some patients in chemotherapy, for example, may feel emotionally affected by the prospects of losing their hair and other physical alterations. In this regard, gender expectations tend to play a role in what doctors assume about men and women with respect to superficiality, but the first ground rule in breaking bad news is that one should never assume anything about an individual patient. The fears associated with family and friends revolve around interpersonal dynamics with others, such as the fear of losing sexual attraction to their significant other, thereby affecting their marriage, or the fear of burdening family members with their problem if they become weakened to the point of hospice care. Last, the fears associated with social and professional life include worries surrounding the loss of one's job, its impact on their financial standing, how they will manage to cover large medical expenses, and the idea of not feeling like a normal part of society. The fears of dying are not universal in nature, but are individual; therefore the key to identifying these fears is going through this list of possible fears and getting the patient to reveal which fear(s) they are experiencing.

# Doctors: Emotional and Psychological Factors

The emotional and psychological factors regulating the effects of giving bad news may vary between health care professionals. One of the most common emotions doctors experience when delivering bad news to patients is the fear of causing the patient emotional and psychological pain. Since pain relief and curative therapy is one of the primary goals of health care, it is understandable that doctors experience irrational feelings of guilt when they are the source of inflicting the immediate reactions of emotional and psychological stress among patients. The ways that doctors experience their own pain vary. Some doctors recall feeling sympathetic pain, which equates to the discomfort of being in the same room with someone under duress.

Health care practitioners also fear the possibility of being blamed through a kind of negative transference in which the patient "shoots the messenger" and cannot, if for only a moment, distinguish between the illness and the doctor's role in causing the pain. For example, if the doctor offers an apology, he or she runs the risk of having this construed as an apology for the doctor's actions rather than as an apology expressed to convey sympathy for the patient's medical predicament as a matter of random chance. If "shooting the messenger" seems irrational from your perspective as a physician, consider your own reaction when someone delivered bad news to you in a non-medical setting. Perhaps you went to a restaurant and became upset with the waiter after learning the restaurant no longer offered your favorite dish. Maybe the price of oil spiked and you expressed disapproval to the gas station attendant. Many doctors know how being blamed feels and eventually, the learned emotional response is to try to avoid it. Unfortunately, avoiding the inevitable result of causing pain ultimately paints the doctor as unsympathetic and only causes further emotional and psychological distress to the patient. Blame also can result from today's expectations in modern medicine, which nurtures the misguided mainstream belief that we can cure anything, so when things go wrong, the doctor must be at fault.

Likewise, doctors tend to flagellate themselves over therapeutic failures, in part because of the reinforced training from medical schools, which focus on reversible or treatable diseases. In Robert Buckman's seminal book, *How to Break Bad News*, the problem of ingrained learning at the educational level indicates a systemic failure that leaves doctors ill-prepared for unexpected turns in disease control. "In all our training, we are taught to deal with a myriad of reversible or treatable conditions ... However, the curriculum is so full of these conditions that there is virtually no teaching on the subject of therapeutic impotence. What do you do when you cannot reverse a disease? The answer, of course, is embodied in the entire discipline of palliative care medicine, in which therapeutic endeavor is not directed at the disease but its symptoms. However, most medical schools and nursing schools do not teach palliative care medicine in the undergraduate program, and as a result, most medical students evolve into physicians who are keen to treat curable conditions, but have little training in what to do with chronic irreversible diseases."

With little training in the handling of incurable disease, doctors who normally exude confidence in their vast professional knowledge may shake the patient's confidence in them by appearing uncertain. Unfortunately, this can directly raise the specter of litigation. According to *The Handbook of Communication in Oncology and Palliative Care*, "A retrospective review of 444 surgical malpractice claims identified inexperience/lack of technical confidence and communication breakdown as the leading system factors behind surgical error." In other words, when the patient's confidence in the physician wanes as a direct result of poor communication, the patient assumes the doctor was responsible for the adverse outcome, not the disease itself.

Given the frequency of lawsuits brought against medical institutions, it should then not be surprising that the fear of the untaught would preclude doctors from seeming more open when it comes to disclosing bad news to a patient. It also explains why medical students evolve into physicians that develop rigid personas and adhere to the guidelines they have learned. The effect to the doctor-patient relationship, of course, becomes counterproductive and provides logical justification for considering communication as a clinical skill and a core component of clinical management. Educational exclusion of this clinical skill incorrectly leads physicians to perceive the skill as optional.

Physicians also retreat emotionally and psychologically from providing communication and emotional support during interviews for fear of inciting a strong emotional response from the patient. In some cases, the mandate comes from the physician's institutional peers who believe it is best practice to avoid upsetting the patient. In doing so, physicians break bad news in such a way that minimizes time spent on communicating information and thereby reduces the patient's emotional response. You may be avoiding your own emotional and psychological discomfort. Are you truly doing what is in the best interest of the patient? In a 2002 medical *Journal of Psycho-Oncology*, a study highlighting audiotapes from 300 cancer patients, which asked a median of 11 questions regarding doctor's responses to emotional cues, only 28 percent of patients reported appropriate empathic responses by their doctors during the clinical interview, while only 72 percent of patients reported appropriate verbal responses by their doctors regarding informational responses. Moreover, providing minimal support to avoid discomfort of an angry emotional response means you run the risk of angering the patient who later finds out that you failed to provide adequate disclosure. In some cases, doctors simply avoid communication to absolve themselves of admitting that they cannot give the patient an exact answer or prognosis. While you may not know the answer to everything, admitting that you do not have the information the patient wants serves to establish an honest relationship and can increase the level of trust in your ability to provide managed care.

The fear of expressing emotion is another emotional and psychological factor that typically minimizes the way health care practitioners communicate to patients. Since logic and reason is a core component of decision-making in the medical profession, many doctors support the notion that an emotionally removed approach fosters sound decision-making and professional behavior. While such an approach may work well for other situations, it rarely works during a doctor-patient interview involving bad news, and often produces the effect of appearing cold-hearted during a time in which the patient is most vulnerable.

Contrary to popular belief, a great many doctors do experience strong emotions but suppress them for the sake of appearing in control, particularly when it comes to patients that remind them of their own personal or family history with a specific illness. To reiterate, in life we are amidst death. No one escapes the primal fear of death as an active agent in the unconscious behaviors of day-to-day living, including doctors. As such, emotional detachment from bad news may begin to settle into the minds of physicians who constantly encounter illness as a means of more effectively dealing with its frequency.

# Culture and Societal Factors

The emotional and psychological effects of bad news may also have roots in the fabric of a given culture or society. Social attitudes in western society place a strong emphasis on materialism, which include financial worth, social status, physical appearance, and so forth, so as one's health situation deteriorates, his or her future prospects for material worth and gain come under threat, creating a sense of outrage toward any causes that would interrupt these goals. Hence, people in western societies may develop a sense of denial when it comes to facing the possibility of death, leaving health care practitioners with the challenge of getting the patient to accept the new reality.

Religion also may play into the social attitude of a culture or society. Western views on religion are now more varied. No longer can someone offering spiritual guidance rely on a uniform belief in order to bring the patient some peace. Thus, the new paradigm for spiritual guidance is to listen to the patients' individualized beliefs and provide healing support tailored to spiritualism as the patient sees it. With social developments over the last 50 years having shifted toward managed care that upholds the patient's right to know his or her health situation, patients have the option of determining how much they want to know, how much information their doctor is allowed disclose to friends and family, and how their treatment plan will unfold.

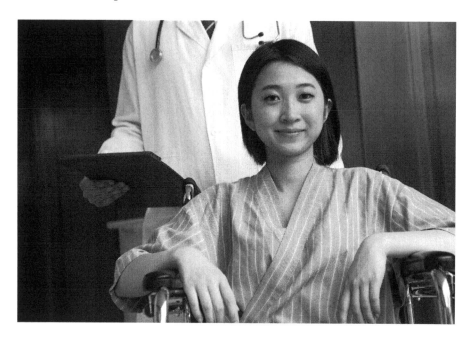

However, as western societies become more ethnically diverse, a greater variety of social attitudes will make it increasingly more difficult to rely on the prevailing attitudes of a given western society. While immigrants begin to adopt the social attitudes of their host country over time, the assimilative process typically takes at least one or two generations. Therefore, first-generation immigrants, while living in western societies, may cling to the social attitudes of their homeland and expect their caregivers to observe said customs. In many Asian, African, and Middle Eastern societies, social attitudes focus more on information disclosure with the patient's family and withholding information from the patient.

To complicate matters, language barriers may impede the quality of care. In a comparative study of acculturated stress, J.W. Berry found that foreigners with limited English had significantly worse access to care and health status compared to other English-proficient foreigners. In Sondra Theiderman's book, *Profiting in America's Multicultural Marketplace*, reluctance on the part of caregivers to notice or observe cultural differences in patients stem from several fears, which include the fear of seeming racist, the fear of perpetuating stereotypes, and the fear of confusing the patient. A suggested remedy to the language and culture barrier is the use of translators to increase communication and find out what social attitudes may guide the information exchange so that the quality of care improves. A 2004 report from *The Journal of General Internal Medicine* concluded that patients who used interpreter services had a greater uptake of recommended preventative services at an estimated cost of $279 per case. For the sake of ease, we recommended that health care practitioners form professional relationships with local interpreter services for on-call activities as needed.

# Initial Patient Reactions to Serious Medical News

In 1969, Elizabeth Kubler-Ross pioneered her landmark book, *On Death and Dying*, which catalyzed the growth and development of palliative care and psychological oncology, thereby changing cancer care practice in North America and most European countries. The Kubler-Ross model for the dying process has since become the study of most academic psychology, psychiatry, social work, and nursing institutions. Her model classifies the dying process into five stages following stability: denial, anger, bargaining, depression, and acceptance. Since the publication of *On Death and Dying*, researchers have incorporated two additional stages: shock (or immobilization) and testing.

*Figure 1. The Kubler-Ross Extended Grief Cycle*

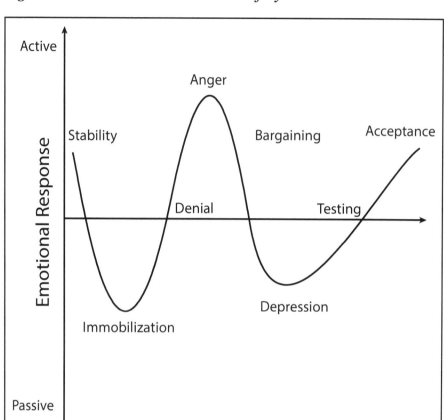

In the shock stage, patients may experience symptoms of physical and emotional paralysis at hearing bad news. Initially, it may appear as if there is no reaction at all to the news. The person may show outward signs of cognition, but they have internally pushed away the news, so the physician may need to reiterate the news several times. Internal shock usually gives way to visible shock, whereby the practitioner may observe physical reactions such as paling of the skin or shortness of breath. The next stage following shock is denial. Symptoms of denial occur when the patient tries to avoid dealing with the situation. The expression of humor may be a symptom of denial or a way of coping, depending on the physician's assessment of the patient's long-term behaviors. In denial, the patient simply blocks or regards the information as untrue and resumes acting as if nothing in their life has changed. Patients frequently become stuck in one phase of the Kubler-Ross grief cycle. The danger presented here is that it prevents them from moving toward the acceptance phase. Since the health care practitioner cannot formulate a management plan until the patient has reached the acceptance phase, the goal of this process is to assist the patient in reaching the final phase (acceptance). While the patient must move through the phases at their own pace, there comes a point where they need to move on toward the next phase.

If your patient appears stuck in denial for an unhealthy period, you can move them out of the denial phase by deliberating provoking the anger phase through a frank discussion of what the future will look like for the patient. Remind them that their situation is not fair and legitimize their anger by demonstrating your own anger over the situation. Symptoms commonly observed in the anger stage include a frustrated outpouring of bottled up emotion. It is at this stage that physicians are most commonly blamed, albeit indiscriminately. Patients become furious and tend to verbalize the question, "Why me?" followed by anger at others simply for not being affected. The key to handling the anger phase is to avoid reacting in any way that appears defensive or argumentative and let the emotional storm run its course. Support the patients' anger; let them direct their anger toward you. By doing otherwise, you run the risk of letting the patient slip back into the denial stage.

During the bargaining stage, the patient is seeking an alternative way out of the situation. Emotional expressions of hope that the doctor can work to reverse the diagnosis become symptomatic at this stage. In looking for signs of hope, the patient may ask about alternative therapies and experimental drugs. When patients enter the bargaining phase, do not offer false hope. Instead, offer practical approaches to treatment and leave the discussion about alternative therapies for after the patient has reached the acceptance phase. When bargaining recedes, the patient inevitably sinks into a mild or severe state of depression. In this state, they only envision the worst and internalize the feeling. Refusing help and general loss of interest earmark the symptoms commonly observed in the depression phase. In this phase, they have shifted the blame from external causes (such as the doctor who gave them the news) to internal causes (such as their own actions). The most common symptoms of depression include loss of appetite, loss of happiness, disordered sleep patterns, disordered physical activity, exhaustion and fatigue, feelings of worthlessness, lack of concentration, and thoughts of dying or suicide. The key to managing the depression phase is to emphasize the positive and reassure them that they will not be alone or abandoned through the course of their illness trajectory while facilitating movement toward the testing phase with a referral for a special counseling service.

During the testing stage, the patient begins to seek realistic goals. They may seek activities designed for the sole purpose of keeping themselves out of depression. Patients often seek such activities with the help of family and friends, as well as professionals who specialize in helping people rediscover their reasons for living. As these activities provide reasons for moving forward and work to restabilize the patient, they near the final stage of the Kubler-Ross model: acceptance. In the acceptance phase, the patient is ready and actively involved in the health management plan and decision-making process. Common symptoms of acceptance include taking ownership of actions, making adjustments in those actions, and increased happiness. The health care practitioner's role during the acceptance phase is to monitor their behavior to make sure they do not regress back into the previous stages.

## Emotional Reactions

During your observation of the grief cycle, it is important to know the difference between initial reactions to bad news and stages of grief. A patient's initial reactions to serious medical news are the symptoms demonstrated within each stage and remain in accordance with behaviors consistent to the person's character. If your patient demonstrates a low level of anger in the anger phase, the current stage of grief may be more difficult to identify. In some cases, the patient may experience simultaneous emotional reactions (ex. denial and anger at the same time). If so, which stage of grief are they experiencing? The only way to know is to continue observing their behaviors until the predominant symptom emerges. Emotional reactions also allow doctors to establish a framework for emotional tendencies because they serve as a reliable indicator for how their patient handled crisis in the past, as well as their general disposition. Establishing framework for emotional tendencies then allows the doctor to formulate an approach for future consultations where the doctor may further disclose bad news.

Just as it may be difficult to distinguish between the stages of grief, it may also be difficult to distinguish between two different emotional reactions. Fear and anxiety are two emotional expressions that doctors frequently confuse. While anxiety exists as a general feeling of discomfort without specific trigger events, fear tends to be a more specific feeling of discomfort triggered by an equally specific event. Clinical phobias, for instance, relate to a fear, both specific and disproportionate in nature, with specific trigger events (the fear of closed spaces, the fear of flying, the fear of death, etc.). Anxieties, by contrast, tend to be more chronic and may take longer to resolve. So where does fear and anxiety exist in the Kubler-Ross model? The answer lies in conducting an exploration into their trigger mechanisms. For example, suppose you ask the patient to describe what they are experiencing and discover that this patient's family has a high incidence of cancer, having lost a mother and two aunts, and the patient expresses worry over his or her three children. You immediately know the reaction is fear, as the trigger event is specific, and that the fear probably relates to anger at the prospects of their children growing up without them or the children developing cancer themselves. The four steps to identifying these ambiguous states of emotion are:

- Identifying the root cause of the ambiguous state
- Acknowledging the emotion driving the reaction
- Offering information relevant to allaying the emotion
- Offering empathic support after the state is no longer ambiguous

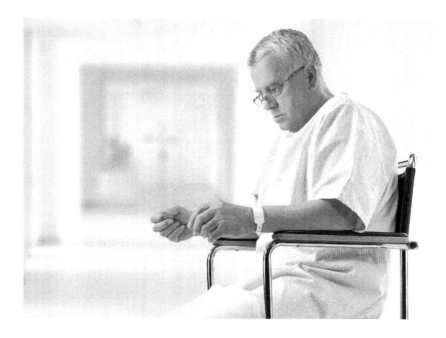

## Three-Stage Model of the Dying Process

While the Kubler-Ross model conceptualizes the stages of the grief cycle, the grief cycle is broken into three categories. The first stage includes the patient's initial reactions of shock, anger, denial, and bargaining. The second stage, known as the chronic stage, encapsulates the patient's depressive experiences, which occur after they have already adjusted to the prospect of dying. They know recovery is not possible, but the possibility of death remains at a distance on the illness trajectory. The chronic stage is marked with the same emotions from the initial stage but with peaks and valleys of diminished intensity — the very characteristics of depression. In rare cases, however, emotional intensity remains high until the final stage has ended. In the final stage, the patient reaches acceptance, characterized by signs of normal communication and little distress.

# Patients' Emotional Needs After Hearing Bad News

Patients who report dissatisfaction with their professional caregiver's communication during a clinical interview cite a common reason: the caregiver has failed to meet their emotional needs. Ironically, the patient will rarely communicate his or her psychosocial needs to the physician despite its importance to the patient. Likewise, physicians pay minimal attention to patients' psychosocial and health-related quality of life concerns. For example, a 2004 report in *Psycho-Oncology* reported that, "Palliative outpatients receiving chemotherapy are less likely to initiate discussion of emotional functioning and daily activities than they are to initiate discussion of aspects of their disease and treatment." The three most common emotional needs reported by patients include the need for control, the need to be heard by their physician, and the need for assurance. While other parts of this book will focus on identifying and responding to emotional cues, this section focuses solely on causality and cursory definitions of emotional need.

## *The Need for Control*

The need for control stems from psychological factors relating back to the initial loss of control felt by the patient after receiving their diagnosis. The Kubler-Ross model illustrates not only the cycle of grief experienced by patients after hearing serious medical news, but also demonstrates the process by which a patient circles back to a state of stability and control. As previously mentioned, society's shift away from a paternalistic approach to managed care toward a patient-centered approach has meant that patients expect the doctor to formulate a management plan according to the patient's own psychosocial agenda. In other words, the patient wants control of information disclosure, choice of treatments, regulation of treatment, whether or not doctors may share the information with others, and so forth. The patient-centered communicator adapts his or her communication in response to the perspectives, feelings, and intentions of others. The Comskil model, discussed in the next few pages, is one such approach to meeting the patient-centered agenda.

## *The Need to be Heard*

The need to be heard likewise stems from patients' desires to formulate their own managed care agenda. This is why the act of listening outweighs technical competence when it comes to patients surveyed for doctor satisfaction. According to a 1984 study by H.B. Beckman in the *Annals of Internal Medicine*, "The average time that a patient is allowed to talk before being interrupted by the physician is 18 seconds, and only 23 percent of patents ever finish their opening statements." Studies further show that when techniques such as repeating the same words patients have used in their communication, patients report increased satisfaction with their physician. What listening confirms to patients is that the doctor is paying attention to their psychosocial needs and plans to incorporate the patient's concerns into the management plan. Responding to emotional reactions with empathic statements also verbalizes what the patient is feeling and affirms listening (see Chapter 3 for further explanation and techniques on using empathic statements).

## The Need for Assurance

The need for assurance relates to the patient's emotional needs regarding his or her worries concerning their future. The range of post-diagnosis emotions may include living with uncertainty, fear of recurrence, concerns over impact on sexuality or body image, employment, finances, and relationship issues. The need for assurance is about searching for hope and allaying specific fears, and the physician needs to address them during the initial clinical interview. Current guidelines for providing assurance recommend that physicians strike a balance between honest disclosure and sustaining hope when they must give bad news to their patients. Even if the physician cannot make assurances, striking a delicate balance guides patients toward integration of the new information within a framework that sustains hope for a better future.

# The Importance of Identifying the Patient's Reactions

By identifying the patient's initial reactions to bad news (i.e. anger, anxiety, fear, etc.), the physician makes the first important assessment as to how the patient has received bad news; that is, whether or not the reactions are typical or atypical, normal or pathological. The Kubler-Ross model of the grief cycle is a physician's barometer for determining this type of assessment. If the patient reactions become long-term behavior patterns, the physician must identify the behaviors as either adaptive or maladaptive to the patient's care. Behaviors can be adaptive or maladaptive behaviors depending on how long it takes the patient to progress toward activities associated with the acceptance phase. For the sake of assessing long-term behaviors, it becomes important to begin identifying the patient's reactions during the initial interview in order to track the patient's progress along the stages of grief. Chapter 3 will discuss in further detail how to determine whether a patient has adopted adaptive or maladaptive behaviors. Here, we identify three criteria for what constitutes normal behavior.

To meet the criteria for normal behavior, a patient's behavior must be fixable, socially acceptable, and demonstrate adaptability. Since a wide range of reactions and behaviors are common at the outset of receiving bad news, physicians should resist the mistake of hastily attempting to classify the initial reactions as adaptive or maladaptive. While heightened levels of emotional temperature such as crying, humor, or shouting are understandable and socially accepted reactions considering the situation, certain reactions do fall outside the norms of social acceptance. For example, if the patient attempts to cause harm to the nurses and doctors after receiving bad news, this may present itself as an extreme form of blaming the messenger. While socially unacceptable, this type of violent anger still corresponds to the stages of grief. However, if expressed as a long-term behavior it becomes maladaptive to the patient's treatment and the physician's goals of care. When reactions do occur, the physician immediately must begin to assess whether or not it contributes to adaptability. In other words, if the initial reactions show no indication of increasing patient distress or causing future disruptions to patient care, then it has the potential of evolving into an adaptive behavior. If the initial reaction has the potential to disrupt care and increase the patient's distress, then it has the potential of evolving into a maladaptive behavior. If the reaction indicates the potential for maladaptive behavior, the physician must assess if the potentially maladaptive behavior is fixable. If intervention methods such as counseling are available, the behavior is fixable. If no interventions appear adequate, the behavior may not be fixable.

# CASE STUDY

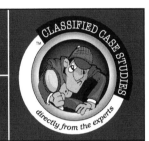

**Name: Dr. Deanna Attai**
**Title: Board Certified Surgeon**
**State: California**

**Excerpt Taken From:** Cancer Emotional Well Being.com, *Interview with Breast Surgeon Dr. Deanna Attai, Part 1*

"There is no doubt in my mind that a frantic life and mind will lead to chronic inflammation; chronic stress and inflammation can affect many systems, including the immune system and the mechanisms by which our bodies repair damage. Keeping the body and mind as calm, rested, and nourished as possible just makes sense to keep damage to a minimum. I do believe that if the depression or "negative" emotion becomes more constant or interferes with treatment or recovery, that specific treatment (which may be as simple as having someone to talk to) can be a huge help. Constant fear and depression may lead to either a suppression of the immune response and/or constant "state of alert," which can feed into the chronic inflammation cycle. When I diagnose my patients with breast cancer, the patient and family members experience a new level of stress on many levels.

I think one of the most important things is that the family tries to come together for the patient. Listen to her, just support her, and if you are not sure what to do, ask her what she wants or needs. Education is important. I encourage patients to bring a family member to their appointments so everyone has the same information. Then everyone needs to breathe, relax, and take some time to let the diagnosis and information sink in before jumping into a plan of action. Going forward, continue to remember that the patient is the one with the disease. While the whole family is affected, keeping the patient's wishes and best interest front and center will help. However, that is often easier said than done; normal roles and routines are terribly disrupted, and asking for help — whether help with normal chores and errands or help in terms of therapy and counseling — is important for the patient and the family. I find that providing direct and accurate information helps a lot, [as well as] encouraging patients to ask questions, allowing them to discuss their fears, and providing them with outlets (referral to a therapist, info on supportive measures, network of complementary therapists, etc.)."

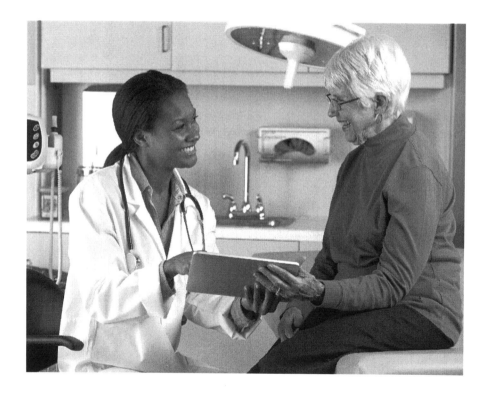

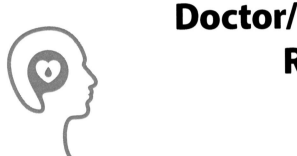

# Chapter 2

# Establishing Doctor/Patient Rapport

stablishing doctor/patient rapport is the first step in clinical communication with patients, and it begins from the moment you meet your patients. Any misstep in the earliest stage of the interview can lead to a relationship that founders and leaves the patient dissatisfied or uncooperative. High-functioning doctor-patient relationships typically exhibit three characteristics: mutual attention, positivity, and coordination. A clinical relationship has reached a state of mutual attention, positivity, and coordination when both parties are listening to what the other person is saying, showing interest, productively exchanging information, moving forward in non-combative ways, and working together toward an agreed-upon goal. In this chapter, we will define the objectives of the clinical relationship, starting with the basic structure of the clinical communication exchange.

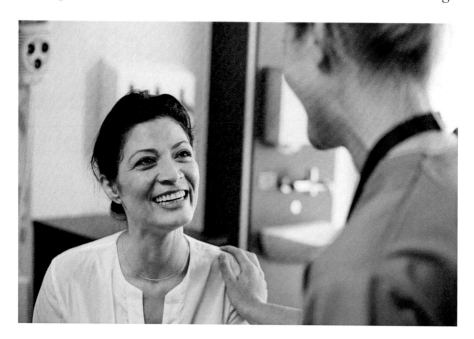

# Theoretical Models of Communication Skills Training

In May 1999, leaders and representatives from major medical education and professional organizations attended an invitational conference to create a consensus on a coherent set of theoretical models for clinical communication with patients. From that conference, these leaders created the seven models that currently help train medical students on how to open a consultation, deliver bad news, and direct patient behavior toward a positive clinical agenda that satisfies the patient's needs and the physician's treatment goals. While each theoretical model only highlights major emphasis points, this book will elaborate further on specific process tasks of clinical interviews in later chapters.

The purpose of these theoretical models is to provide some structure to the communication strategies outlined in this book. Once you have learned the finer details of communication, the knowledge can be reflowed into any of these theoretical models according to their design and applied in earnest. However, with the exception of the Comskil model, researchers designed these models with the intention of dealing with the initial clinical encounter, rather than ongoing palliative or hospice care. Since many health care practitioners must deliver bad news beyond the initial interview and along the illness trajectory (such as telling patients that treatments are not working), you will recognize components of the Comskil model throughout this book. The seven theoretical models are:

- The Bayer Institute for Healthcare Communication E4 Model
- The Three-Function Model
- The Calgary-Cambridge Observation Guide
- The Patient-Centered Clinical Method
- The SEGUE Framework
- The Four-Habits Model
- The Comskil Model

## The Bayer Institute E4 Model

Physicians typically use the E4 model for situations (such as drug addiction) whereby the behaviors may have directly caused the medical problem. The E4 model aims to assist in positive behavioral change while maximizing the patient's confidence in changing behavior. To accomplish these goals, the E4 model suggests providing information in small doses called "chunking" in order to set the agenda. This is important because errors and lapses in memory can drastically alter a patient's understanding of their situation and negatively impede your clinical goals of care. A 2003 report in the *Journal of the Royal Society of Medicine* indicated that patients forget 40 to 80 percent of medical information provided by health care practitioners immediately following consultation. In essence, the greater the amount of information presented, the lower the amount of recall, with almost half the amount of recall being incorrect. To achieve its goals, the E4 (or four E's) recommends four steps.

- Step 1: Engage
- Step 2: Empathize
- Step 3: Educate
- Step 4: Enlist

The first step in the E4 model is to engage the patient by eliciting the patient's story and listening for their understanding of the illness. Taking the patient's account becomes essential to forming any patient-centered agenda because it enables the physician to distinguish between what the body is experiencing from what the person (i.e. emotional component) is experiencing. To elicit the patient's story, the doctor starts by saying, "Tell me everything that occurred when you began experiencing this problem." After the patient gives the account of the problem, the second step in the E4 model is to demonstrate empathy by calling attention to the patient's feelings and values, which signals to the patient that you have listened to their story. Following an empathic response, the third step is to educate the patient by answering questions he or she indirectly posed during their account. At the end of these clinical explanations, the physician should always check for understanding by directly asking the patient if he or she has understood the explanations and their potential implications. In the final step of the E4 model, the physician enlists the patient's participation in the decision-making process and encourages continued involvement. Physicians trained under the E4 model receive ratings on the Likert scale for their performance of each step. The ratings take into account the physician's measure of empathy, patient reactions to the physician's methods, and several interactional items. The Bayer Institute has based the E4 model on the Prochaska and DiClemente stages of change model, which delineates the stages the patient must go through in order to achieve maintenance of desirable behavior. For more information on the E4 model or training, contact the Institute for Healthcare Communication at **http://healthcarecomm.org**.

## The Three-Function Model

Medical schools and institutions use the three-function model as a means of helping health care practitioners improve their interviewing skills with patients. The three-function model identifies three essential components. They are:

- Building the relationship
- Assessing the patient's problem
- Managing the patient's problem

In order to build the relationship, this model emphasizes the use of empathy, support, and respect as initial physician responses to a patient's emotions. In Steven Cole's book, *The Medical Interview,* the author cites empathic appreciation of emotion as the single most important quality of relationship building, manifested in five specific responses: reflection, legitimization, personal support, partnership, and respect. In this model, the physician assesses the patient's problem through nonverbal listening, asking open-ended questions, facilitating discussion, and clarifying information. Chapter 3 will discuss listening techniques that acknowledge the patient's responses in further detail.

After assessing the problem, the physician then manages the patient's problem by checking the patient's understanding, recommending a treatment plan, and checks the patient's willingness to proceed. The three-function model also offers categorized communication behaviors that can operationalize the interview process for greater communication from the opening dialogue, through the discussion, to the closing comments. For further reading on the three-function model, consult Steven Cole's book, *The Medical Interview*.

## *The Calgary-Cambridge Observation Guide*

The Calgary-Cambridge observation guide — developed by Suzanne Kurtz, Jonathan Silverman, John Benson, and Juliet Draper —integrates both content and process where other conceptual frameworks may compartmentalize them. For example, while "building the relationship" exists as a first step in the three-function model, the Calgary-Cambridge observation guide structures "building the relationship" as an ongoing and active function during the implementation of five subroutines, which include:

- Initiating the session
- Gathering information
- Physical examination
- Explanation and planning
- Closing the session

Figure 2 is a visual model of the Calgary Cambridge observation guide. See Appendix C for the more advanced version of this model. For further information on this model, go to **www.skillscascade.com/handouts/CalgaryCambridgeGuide.pdf** or access the Calgary-Cambridge pages at **www.gp-training.net**.

*Figure 2. The Calgary-Cambridge Observation Guide*

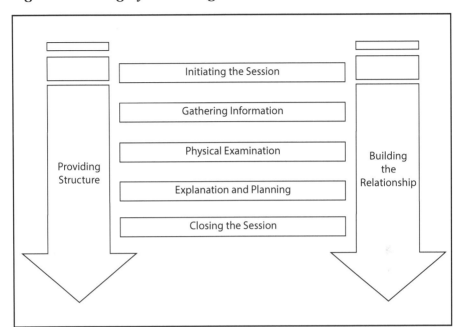

# The Patient-Centered Clinical Method

The Patient-Centered Clinical Method explores six steps.

## Step 1

**Explore the disease and the illness experience.** While doctors focus on the identification, treatment, and prevention of disease, patients focus on the experience of the disease. To explore the experience of the illness, the physician must get the patient's ideas as to what he or she thinks is wrong, listen to the patient's fears about the problem, verbalize what the patient expects from the physician, and explain the effect of the illness upon functioning.

## Step 2

**Understand the whole person.** This means becoming aware of cultural influences guiding the patient's beliefs, behaviors, responses, and expectations in order to assess the patient's response to the illness and therapy. By understanding the whole person, we can understand the impact of an illness on the patient's daily life and more effectively tailor a treatment regimen to fit the patient's circumstances.

## Step 3

**Negotiate with patients to find common ground.** Sometimes in a doctor-patient relationship, both parties have a different agenda in mind for treatment. Under this step, the physician can align the patient's agenda with his or her own by reaching an agreement on the nature of the problem, establishing goals and priorities of treatment, and identifying roles for the clinician and patient.

## Step 4

**Incorporate health promotion and disease prevention.** Step 4 serves a retroactive step. Achieving an understanding of the whole person in Step 2 facilitates the possibility of implementing health promotion and disease prevention strategies. The negotiation of health promotion and disease prevention begins as a discussion in Step 3. The goals of this discussion may include health enhancement suggestions (such as an exercise program), risk reduction strategies (such as discontinuing an unhealthy behavior), clinical recommendations for early detection (such as monitoring), and working to change or reverse the effects of the disease (such as life extension therapies).

## Step 5

**Describe ways to enhance the doctor-patient relationship.** In community-based primary care practice, you see the same patients continually over time. The patient-centered clinical method encourages the practice of therapeutic attributes such as empathy, respect, positive regard, reciprocity; the sharing of power and control; the recognition of differences; knowing the patient's strengths, weaknesses, biases and emotional triggers; and the frequency of transference and countertransference in the relationship (i.e. the unconscious agendas both parties bring to the relationship).

## Step 6

**Develop realistic expectations about the relationship.** Letting the patient know that you cannot address all concerns or fix every problem prevents the patient from attaining any false hope. This step is a reminder that doctor-patient relationships gradually build over time rather than during the first interview alone.

*Figure 3. The Patient-Centered Clinical Method*

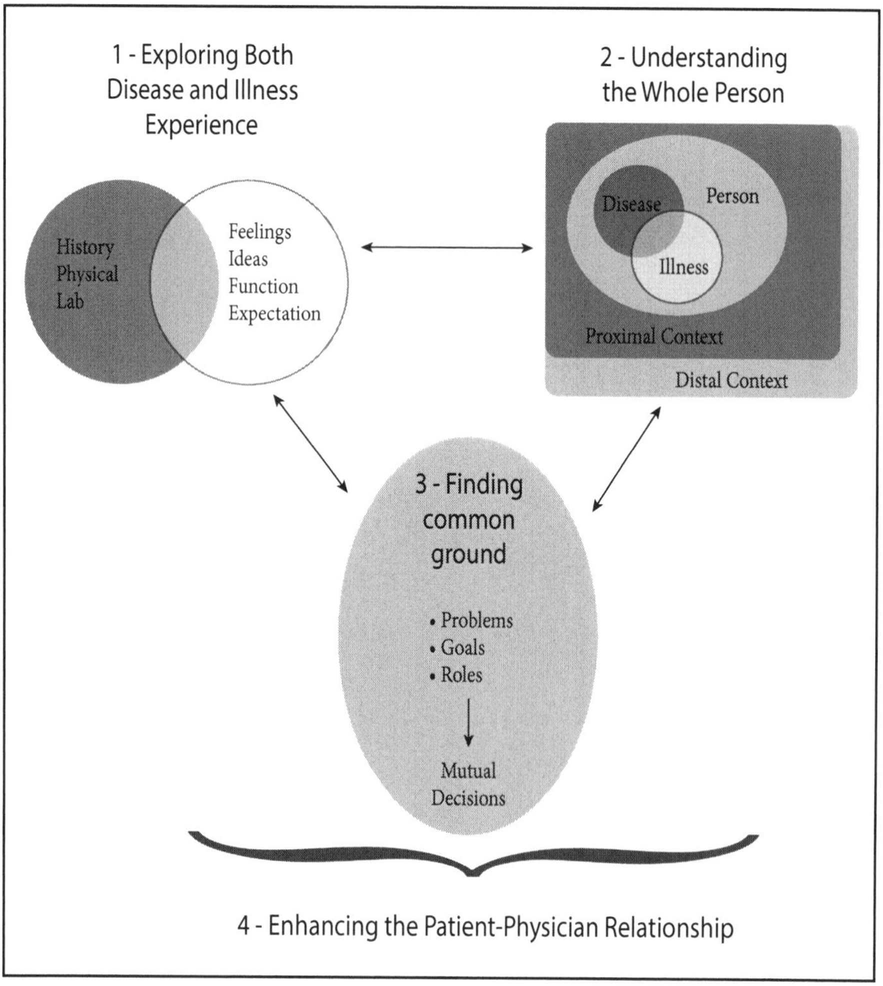

1 - Exploring Both Disease and Illness Experience

History Physical Lab

Feelings Ideas Function Expectation

2 - Understanding the Whole Person

Disease   Person

Illness

Proximal Context

Distal Context

3 - Finding common ground

• Problems
• Goals
• Roles

Mutual Decisions

4 - Enhancing the Patient-Physician Relationship

## The SEGUE Framework

The SEGUE framework is an acronym for a five-step clinical encounter. A recent survey indicated that it is the most widely-used structure for communication skills teaching and assessment in U.S and Canadian medical schools. For the SEGUE checklist listing the tasks for each step, see Appendix B.

- Set the stage
- Elicit information
- Give information
- Understand the patient's perspective
- End the encounter

## The Four-Habits Model

The four-habits model consists of various communication tasks that make up each habit, organized into an interrelated grouping of skills, techniques, and payoffs. For example, if the physician fails to address the patient's concerns at the beginning of the encounter, the physician risks creating false hypotheses, as well as misplaced empathy and support. For further details on the four-habits model, see Appendix A.

### Habit 1

**Invest in the beginning.** This habit places emphasis on the first few moments of the medical encounter, using the first few seconds to establish a welcoming atmosphere to give the patient a sense of safety. Habit 1 stresses adaptations in voice tone, language level, and posture to convey the clinician's attentiveness in response to the patient.

### Habit 2

**Elicit the patient's perspective.** This habit helps determine the reasons for the patient's visit. Habit 2 recommends three strategies for eliciting the patient's perspective: the use of open-ended questions (ex: "Tell me about the pain you've been having"), the use of linguistic devices called "continuers," (ex: "uh huh," "I see," "Go on," "Tell me more"), and nonverbal behaviors (silence, vertical head shaking, engaged listening posture).

## Habit 3

**Demonstrate empathy.** This habit stresses the action of identifying hidden emotions that patient's reveal through verbal hints, and seizing "windows of opportunity" for responding to patients' emotions. When responding to a potential empathic opportunity, habit 3 recommends the use of continuers in habit 2 to encourage the expression of emotion.

## Habit 4

**Invest in the end.** This habit requires information sharing. The tasks required for habit 4 include delivering diagnostic information (giving good news, bad news, or no news), encouraging patients to participate in future decision-making, negotiating treatment plans, and probing for adherence.

## *The Comskil Model*

The Memorial Sloan-Kettering Cancer Center developed the Comskil model as a way to evaluate skills taught in clinical communication training. Among the models previously mentioned, the Comskil model is the only framework that conceptualizes ongoing patient-doctor communication beyond the initial interview with the patient. The Comskil model addresses communication challenges of continuous care, the skills necessary to meet these challenges, and methods to assess communication skills training. For the training evaluation model, see Appendix E. The core components that comprise the Comskil model are:

- **Goals** — the desired outcome of the situation

- **Strategies** — plans that direct patient behavior toward the desired outcome

- **Skills** — discrete methods to achieve strategies

- **Process Tasks** — dialogues and nonverbal behaviors that create an environment for effective communication

- **Cognitive Appraisals** — hypotheses formed about the patient's hinted agenda and needs

*Figure 4. The Comskil Model*

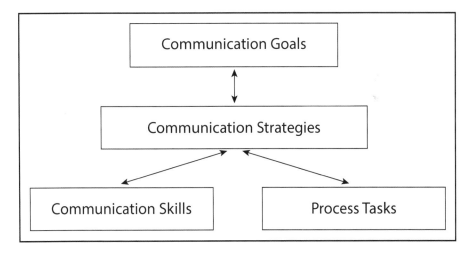

# Communication Goals

The *Handbook of Communication in Oncology and Palliative Care* defines communication goals as the desired outcome of a consultation. In today's patient-centered approach, a communication goal of most consultations focuses on the patient's desired outcome — the patient's goals are the physician's goals. For example, let us suppose you are the oncologist of a patient who, after receiving a cancer diagnosis, expressed worry about their children's welfare. Now let us suppose you discover the patient's family history, which reveals a high incidence of cancer. To discuss this genetic risk with the patient, you set a communication goal. The communication goal in this instance might involve easing the patient's concern for his or her children's welfare. Once you set this goal, you begin to formulate strategies for achieving these desired outcomes by using subtle strategies, skills, process tasks, and cognitive appraisals.

# Communication Strategies

Communication strategies are plans, employed in sequence, that direct patient behavior toward the realization of a communication goal. For example, when we discussed the Bayer Institute E4 model, we mentioned four steps: engage, empathize, educate, and enlist. If a communication goal of the E4 model is to direct the patient's future behavior toward more positive actions, then the communication strategies are the four sequential steps necessary to achieve the outcome.

# Communication Skills

Communication skills are the subtle actions taken within each strategy to elicit further dialogue between the patient and physician. To qualify as a communication skill, the action must be verbal, concrete, teachable, and observable. The *Handbook of Communication in Oncology and Palliative Care* lists six types of clinical communication skills used in a doctor-patient relationship:

- **Consultation framework skills** (skills that set the agenda and invite the patient to explain the purpose of their visit)

- **Empathic communication skills** (skills that recognize, legitimize, and normalize the patient's feelings)

- **Questioning skills** (skills that enable you to get a better understanding of what the patient is feeling)

- **Information organizing skills** (skills that summarize information and make details easier for the patient to digest and recall)

- **Checking skills** (skills that reinforce and confirm the patient's understand of the information you have organized for them)

- **Shared decision-making skills** (skills that explore the patient's desired role in their managed care)

# Process Tasks

Process tasks are specific sets of dialogue and nonverbal actions. Similar to communication skills, they operationalize communication strategies. Process tasks range from basic to complex, and are more specific than communication skills because they describe an exact action taken. For example, paying attention to the specific words used by a patient would be a specific process task that demonstrates the communication skill of empathic listening.

# Cognitive Appraisals

A cognitive appraisal is the process by which a health practitioner makes an internal hypothesis about the patient's hinted agenda and needs.

Once the physician forms a hypothesis, the next step is to explore the hypothesis through further dialogue with the patient. If further dialogue disproves the hypothesis, the physician circles back to strategies meant to uncover the patient's inexplicit agenda until the patient's responses confirm the hypothesis. The Comskil model suggests two types of cognitive appraisals: cues and barriers.

Patient cues describe indirect behaviors used by patients to prompt the doctor for informational or emotional support. In some cases, the patient will ask a question or make a statement that indirectly cues the doctor to provide either information or support. However, because of the indirect nature of cues, the doctor runs the risk of misinterpreting the patient's cue if the hypothesis goes untested through further dialogue. For example, if a patient says, "I'm worried about how my children will react to the news that I have cancer." Immediately, the doctor might form a hypothesis that the patient is looking for assistance in delivering this news, but further exploration of the hypothesis might led the doctor to the realization that the patient is indirectly looking for reassurance that the cancer is not fatal and that the children will not become orphans. Further exploration is necessary; the emotional needs between hypothesis 1 and 2 would require two very different communication strategies.

Patient barriers constitute patient perceptions that impede effective communication. Barriers become increasingly problematic when perceptions remain undisclosed, leaving the physician to either miss the cue or misinterpret their hypothesis. Constant expressions of hesitancy, anxiety, and uncooperative behavior are clear signals of a patient using barriers. The communication skills outlined in this book will help you identify and break through patient barriers.

# Conflicting Goals

As you have probably learned in your experience, the goals *of* the patient may not always align with your goals *for* the patient. As someone of greater knowledge and expertise on the subject of medicine, you may be tempted to discount what the patient wants if you believe it conflicts with your objectives in treating the illness. However, today's patient-centered approach leaves you little choice but to consider the patient's agenda, even if you disagree with it. As such, a physician typically will structure the clinical agenda with four objectives in mind:

- Diagnosis
- Treatment Plan
- Prognosis
- Support

To strike a balance of interests, the patient-centered approach requires eliciting the patient's story of illness while guiding the interview through a process of diagnostic reasoning. The treatment plan requires consideration of the patient's ideas, feelings, and values, weighed against what the physician believes is the best course of action. Delivering prognosis in the patient-centered approach requires careful use of communication skills that bring the patient to acceptance of the new reality while offering a modicum of hope for the future. Support in the patient-centered approach means regarding the physician-patient relationship as a partnership in which you offer consultation but ultimately adhere to the patient's rights and wishes.

# Power Structures in Doctor-Patient Relationships

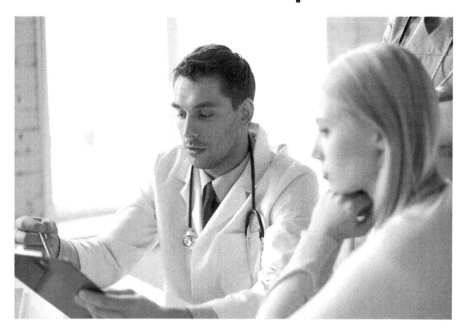

The degree to which doctors have power and influence over their patients can vary from relationship to relationship. In Deborah Roter's book, *Doctors Talking with Patients/Patients Talking with Doctors*, the author lists four different types of power structures.

- High-power doctor/Low-power patient
- Low-power doctor/High-power patient
- High-power doctor/High-power patient
- Low-power doctor/Low-power patient

According to Roter, when a high-power doctor consults a low-power patient, the doctor has assumed a paternalistic approach to care giving. He or she sets the goals of the agenda, does not involve the patient in decision-making, and controls the flow of information given or received. Thus, the patient's values and preferences for managed care have no importance in the relationship. Ironically, the high-power doctor/low-power patient relationship may be the values and preferences of some patients. This is why most researchers recommend that physicians treat every clinical encounter with a patient-centered approach. By showing awareness of the patient's feelings and values, you may conclude what type of power structure the patient is looking for, including the kind where you are asked to have all the power and make all the decisions.

When a low-power doctor consults a high-power patient, the patient expects to set all the goals of the agenda, control the flow of information, and make all the decisions. In this scenario, you are there to carry out the agenda set by the patient and to provide whatever information the patient needs to determine the treatment decisions. When a high-power doctor consults a high-power patient, the doctor and patient mutually set the agenda and collaborate on the decision process. When a low-power doctor consults a low-power patient, roles remain unclear, and participation on both sides is minimal, with few results achieved. When meeting with a patient for the first time, your initial communication goal should be to persuade the patient toward a balanced relationship. If you conclude that the patient desires something other than a balanced relationship, you are obligated to observe the patient's rights.

Roter's book highlights the formative trends that explain why so many high-power doctor/low-power patient relationships exist. "The educational process for physicians begins formally during the premed college years when eligibility for medical school is determined. College undergraduates, determined to enter medical school, show signs and symptoms of what has been termed the premed syndrome — including 'aggressive competitiveness, self-interested pursuit of grades, narrow-minded overspecialization, high anxiety, and more than occasional incidents of academic dishonesty.' These experiences are not inconsequential in molding and selecting people who will ultimately become doctors…" To this end, Roter concludes that the academic orientation of the student's medical schools plays a formative role in how doctors practice medicine, how they view patients, and the types of power structures they are likely to form.

# Nonverbal Communication in the Medical Encounter

Earlier, we defined process tasks as dialogues and nonverbal behaviors that create an effective environment for communication. Studies show that nonverbal exchanges between patients and doctors in the high-power doctor/low-power patient power structure create asymmetrical behaviors within patients. If you demonstrate nonverbal signs of dominance such as invading the patient's proximal space, speaking more authoritatively, or smiling less, the patient is likely to compliment your behavior by showing nonverbal cues of submission. If the patient assumes these nonverbal cues, they are likely to talk less, thereby providing less information, leading you to an incorrect diagnosis. In a 2002 journal of *Psychology and Aging*, Nalini Ambady and Jasook Koo of Harvard University studied the link between health care practitioners patterns of nonverbal behavior and therapeutic efficacy. They discovered that the physician's use of less dominant nonverbal cues can increase the patient's physical and cognitive functioning, whereas more dominant cues sends the patient into physical and cognitive retreat. If Roter's premed syndrome of formative dominance and self-interest bears evidence into the common characteristics of doctors, we may conclude that an overwhelming number of physicians also exhibit nonverbal cues of dominance.

This is not to say that doctors who exhibit signs of dominance never actively assess their patient's nonverbal patient cues. In fact, many doctors who exhibit signs of dominance quite often take a disease-centered approach to diagnosis (i.e. they concentrate on the disease using a variety of methods, including nonverbal cues, to reach a diagnosis). However, in doing so they ignore how their own verbal cues impact the patient's responses, and in some cases, diagnosis. A 2005 study by Jozien Bensing from the *Journal of Nonverbal Behavior* showed that nonverbal behavior can lead to a more accurate diagnosis — with statistical findings that found a direct correlation between positive doctor gaze and consultation length. If Ambady and Koo's study on cognitive function proves anything, dominant physician behavior reduces the level of nonverbal cues the physician may be able to observe. In a 2003 study published in the *Journal of Internal Medicine*, C.H. Griffith showed that patient satisfaction increased when physicians demonstrated friendlier, more positive nonverbal cues such as smiling and using a softer tone of voice. Surgeons demonstrating fewer dominant nonverbal cues with their patients also were reported as less likely to have been sued for medical malpractice.

Rick Nauert of *Psych Central* notes, "The way a patient presents himself may [provide] clues as to whether non-specific symptoms like weight gain, fatigue, and high blood pressure are signals of depression or whether something else may be responsible, like a rare condition such as Cushing syndrome, which may indicate an adrenal tumor. ... Patients, on the other hand, [are] mainly concerned with clues that indicated their place within the doctor-patient relationship. 'Our findings are consistent with research from the social sciences suggesting that doctors' and patients' judgments in the examining room are often complicated and take into account many subtle, unspoken clues,' said senior author Michael Fetters, M.D., M.P.H., M.A."

# Gender Communication Differences Between Health Providers

Research studies reveal measurable differences in the communication style between genders, as well as the influence of gender on doctor-patient rapport. By comparison, female clinicians demonstrate communication styles consistent with patient-centered relationships, whereas male doctors trend toward paternalistic relationships consistent with a more disease-centered approach. However, evidence supports an overall trend toward patient-centered approaches when doctors and patients are the same gender. Patient-centered approaches are more common in male/male or female/female doctor-patient relationships than relationships where the gender pairings are male/female or female/male. These studies — in addition to findings that show equal patient satisfaction for male and female practitioners — conclude that the psychology of role expectation factors into the chosen communication approach of the doctor. For example, while evidence shows that male doctors more frequently adopt patient-centered approaches with male patients, male patients report decreased satisfaction when their male doctors interrupt their description of illness during the consultation. In other words, stereotypical expectation of gender roles correlates to patient satisfaction except when male patients feel dominated by their male doctors. For these reasons, researchers recommend using the communication styles inherent with patient-centered approaches regardless of gender. To establish patient-centered rapport through nonverbal communication, the authors of *Mastering Communication with Seriously Ill Patients* suggest opening the interview with the following nonverbal cues:

- Squarely face the patient to indicate interest
- Adopt an open body posture
- Lean toward the patient

- Use eye contact to show attention
- Maintain a relaxed body posture

# Achieving Culturally Sensitive Communication

In the western world, health care practitioners face intercultural challenges that come with ethnic diversity. How a physician handles language barriers and the social customs of ethnically diverse groups may determine the success or failure of a doctor's communication style. Culturally sensitive communication requires considerations of context. According to the *Handbook of Communication in Palliative Care*, when a cultural encounter shows low context, communication can be task-oriented, straightforward, and unambiguous. If a cultural encounter shows high context, communication is indirect with large amounts of meaning embedded in spoken, written, or nonverbal communication.

On the subject of high context cultural communication, Katharina Manassis writes, "It is important not to ridicule the patient's beliefs, since this does less harm to those beliefs than it does to the physician's ability to provide effective medical care. It is unreasonable to expect a physician to learn every aspect of every culture…" However, "It is essential for the physician to discover the patient's illness model and compare it to his or her own. Specific areas of comparison include beliefs about etiology, onset of symptoms, pathophysiology, course of illness (including its severity and the patient's anticipated sick role), and treatment expectations… Harwood provided an example of this approach in his paper about Puerto Rican patients' illness beliefs. Illness is believed to result from an imbalance of 'hot' and 'cold' foods (not based on the foods' actual temperature), and treatment consists of taking a 'hot' or 'cold' medication to remedy the imbalance. Thus, a patient may stop taking penicillin (a 'hot' medication) if he or she develops diarrhea (a sign of too much 'heat'). The solution lies in getting the patient to take the penicillin with fruit juice, which is 'cold,' to neutralize the excess 'heat.' This approach is called 'reframing' so that it more closely matches the patient's beliefs and values."

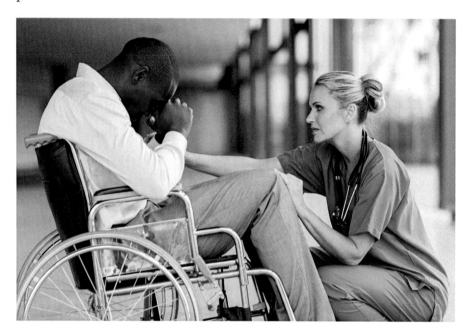

As a general reference, European countries typically engage in low-context communication while Asian, Arab, and African countries engage in high-context communication. High-context situations tend to stress demonstration of respect, and nonverbal customs. It also emphasizes the relation of things and people, and blurs the line between professional and personal life. When your patient is an immigrant or a foreigner, determine the cultural context (high or low) as early as possible. If the situation appears in high context, your communication style should strive to:

- Recognize any participants in the decision-making process besides the patient (such as family or friends)
- Strive for mutual respect among participants

- Clarify the roles of all participants
- Address any rising level of distrust, role conflict, dissatisfaction within the relationship power structure, or miscommunication

The final bullet point on this list brings us to the topic of ambiguity. The use of ambiguity is appropriate for high-context, culture-specific medical situations where you must reveal bad news. In some cultures, patients do not want bad news directly revealed to them, so it is customary to lead the discussion with ambiguity. For example, you might give the patient the option of pursuing or derailing the conversation by asking an open-ended question such as, "What do you think is happening to you?" If the patient confirms what you already know about their prognosis, you may transition the conversation further into specificity. Beware the pitfalls of ambiguity in high-context situations. Incorporating the use of ambiguity as a culture-specific communication skill may create miscommunication. The most effective use of ambiguity is to compress the meaning in your communication by using metaphors. Metaphors are high context stories that allow the listener the opportunity to search for hidden meaning. For example, in the 2012 film, *Life of Pi*, the main character, the son of an Indian zookeeper, tells an allegorical story of his shipwreck at sea. When the listener, a European, discovers that Pi has rearranged key facts, he asks Pi why he changed parts of the story, not realizing that Pi told the story in high context because the events of the shipwreck were too painful for him to speak of aloud. When speakers compress high-context stories through metaphor, the speaker reveals facts through subtext. In other words, they have expressed something without directly verbalizing it. Therefore, in order to communicate in high-context situations, you will need to develop four skills: the ability to recognize the context, the ability to use and understand ambiguous language, the ability to recognize miscommunication caused by ambiguity, and the ability to clarify the miscommunication.

# How to Facilitate the Initial Meeting with a Patient

When meeting a patient for the first time, the importance of getting off to a good start cannot be understated. The first step is finding an appropriate medical setting to discuss bad news. As a general ground rule, physicians should always disclose bad news in person. According to a study published by Stuart Lind and Mary Jo DelVecchio in the *Journal of Clinical Oncology*, 23 percent of patients tabbed for a clinical study on cancer diagnosis reported that their doctors told them over the phone. "Patients told over the telephone or in the recovery room were more likely to describe the telling in negative terms and less likely to describe their doctors as being helpful in understanding their illness than those told in a doctor's office or in their hospital bed," reported Lind and DelVecchio. "Patients who were especially distressed by how they were told the diagnosis often failed to resolve their anger toward their physician."

Consider the experience of Patient No. 48 from this study: "The doctor telephoned to say, 'The bad news is you have a tumor. The good news is that we think [the problem] is meningioma, which means it is easy to get to.' Meanwhile, I am standing there with the phone and my mouth down to the floor, and asking him if I could come in to meet with him. He said, 'Well, [we could meet] next Tuesday.' It still amazes me that that person could do that."

Patient No. 54 described a similar telephone experience. "So he said, 'Oh, by the way, we have a tumor clinic here. We have decided what you really need is a double radical mastectomy, and we will give you beautiful implants.' This is on the phone. So I said, 'Look, I don't care about implants; I want my life.' I'm very outraged at the way he told me all of this over the phone."

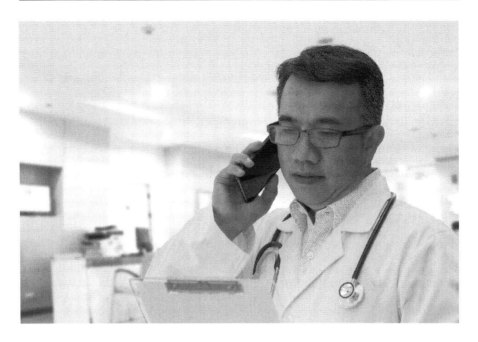

Always deliver bad news in a traditional medical setting such as the doctor's office or hospital room. When patients are not present, contact them by phone and tell them you would like to schedule a clinical interview to discuss their situation. When the patient arrives, seek out a separate office or an interview room. If you are dealing with an in-patient scenario and no such room is available, turn off televisions, lower the bedrail to remove physical barriers, offer to help the patient sit in a chair, and draw the curtains to give the patient a sense of privacy. In either case, always pay attention to your body language, assume normal courtesies such as a formal greeting and handshake, if possible, and ask the patient how he or she is feeling. If the patient responds that they are not feeling well, and the need for the interview is imperative, lead with a statement that acknowledges their current state, and promise that what you have to say will only take a few minutes. If the news requires a longer discussion, ask them for a few minutes, and offer to come back to finish the discussion when they are feeling better.

Once you have secured a proper setting, ask the patient if he or she is comfortable, then sit down if possible, place both feet on the ground, face the patient, and begin the interview by making a welcoming statement. A proper welcoming statement establishes your name, your role as their health care provider, the purpose of the interview, and the time limits of the interview. If family or friends are present, ask the patient if you would like them to stay or have the discussion in private. Completing these process tasks lets the patient know that you have their interests at heart and indicates your intention to facilitate a discussion that considers their agenda.

After your welcoming statement, the next step is to find out what the patient already knows about the illness. Physicians can phrase the question in any number of ways, including:

- How serious do you think the problem is?
- How much has this problem worried you?
- Why do you think the previous doctor sent you to me?
- What do you think about the symptoms you have
  been experiencing?

Listening to the patient's perspective of the medical situation will indicate how far you have to close the gap between reality and their expectation. If they say that they do not know anything, yet the medical record indicates that the previous doctor spoke with them about the problem, assess their emotional position along the Kubler-Ross grief cycle, as they may be traversing along the denial stage. If so, refer to the records and ask them if they remember the previous conversation — it may jar them out of denial or reveal that they were testing you to compare your clinical opinion with another.

When listening, take note of the words used to tell their story. Vocabulary will indicate the level of clinical terminology (or "med-speak") the patient can understand and how much you can use in giving your description of the problem. If they substitute medical terms with basic language, you know that you will have to speak the same way. For example, if a patient describes a metastatic screen as tests the doctors performed to see if the problem spread to other body parts, you know that the patient prefers the use of plain language that is easy to understand. If you ignore the patient's use of plain language and proceed to throw technical terms at them, you run the risk of confusing the patient, and angering them if they later discover the problem and wonder why you did not tell them earlier. Conversely, if the patient uses vocabulary that demonstrates a high use and understanding of clinical terminology, you may proceed to speak in that language. The key skill in this scenario is recognizing the level of understanding, and developing the skill of translating technical or complex explanations into plain language if necessary.

Once you have heard their story, ask them if they would like to discuss the details of the diagnosis, even if the details may indicate something more serious than they anticipated. If they prefer not to discuss the diagnosis, respect their wishes, say you would be happy to have the conversation later if they change their mind, and move on to discussing the treatment plan. If the patient signals consent to inform, the next step is sharing the information as a way of aligning their expectations with reality. The way to align the patient with reality is to first restate what the patient has said, using the same words they used. Not only does this tell the patient that you have listened, it gives you an opportunity to correct misperceived aspects of the problem or instill the patient with confidence that they have a high level of understanding.

As mentioned in our explanation of the E4 model, patient information recall increases when physicians provide details in small doses called chunking. To achieve this effect, speak slowly, offer pauses, allowing the patient to respond, and divide your explanations by asking if the patient understands the information segment covered. Checking reception frequently confirms how much the patient understands, gives the patient another opportunity to speak, reduces a sense of powerlessness brought on by a potentially frightening situation, and demonstrates that you believe their understanding of the problem matters. If the patient verbally or nonverbally shows signs of confusion, consider repeating your major points, using visual aids such as diagrams, or writing down the explanation for them to read later.

After you have provided information and aligned their expectations to reality, ask the patient if they have any concerns. When they finish expressing their concerns, acknowledge this, and allow them to explore those concerns with continuers (see Four-Habits Model). When they have finished voicing their concerns, talk to them about your concerns and propose an agenda that meets both agendas. The physician, therefore, should begin to make a list of the goals for care, and revise according to the feedback provided by the patient. By the time you finish the six-step protocol for getting off to a good start, you will have:

1. Made a welcoming statement
2. Allowed the patient to speak about what they know
3. Aligned their understanding
4. Allowed the patient to voice concerns
5. Proposed an agenda that meets both party's goals
6. Asked for feedback and created a list of goals to incorporate into a mutual agenda

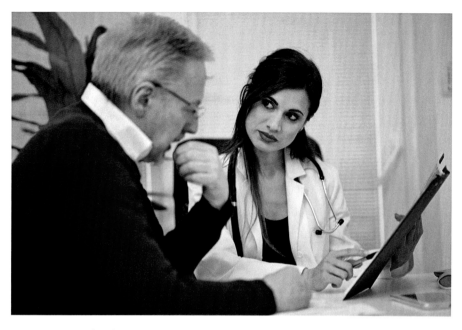

# Determining the Patient's Agenda

In 1999, a study in the *Journal of the American Medical Association* reported that only 28 percent of patients completed their statement of concerns to the doctor during a clinical interview, while the majority of causes for non-completion included no solicitation of concerns or redirection by a closed question. When patients report a lack of interest taken by physicians in tailoring their goals of care to the patient's goals of care, the likely reason is that the physician has not measured the patient's emotional or cognitive data. Cognitive data refers to the intellectual process of thinking, reasoning, and judging. Cognitive data reveals what the patient rationally understands. Emotional data refers to the process of appraising value, creating contextual meaning out of facts, and preparing the brain and body for further action. Since emotions are involuntary responses, emotional function may work at cross-purposes with cognitive functions. For instance, if the patient's emotional data indicates the presence of shock or denial, the emotional data may not only interfere with the patient's cognitive ability to understand and absorb the news, but also with their ability to prepare the brain and body for action. Therefore, in order to determine the patient's agenda, the physician must measure the patient's cognitive and emotional responses by soliciting concerns and then apply aligning techniques to the agenda. Aligning both agendas requires you to:

- Hear the patient's concerns by assessing cognitive and emotional data
- Listen for buried questions and plan to answer them
- Make a list of the patient's concerns and then include them in the topics covered in your conversation
- Negotiate aspects of informed consent and the type of prognostic information the patient desires (i.e. staging details, chances of cure, possible side effects of treatment, survival estimates) and make a note of these preferences for future patient interviews
- Check for cognitive understanding by summarizing the main points of the agenda both parties have agreed to
- Offer emotional support if the emotional data necessitates it

## CASE STUDY

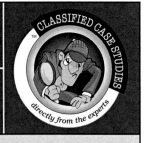

**Name:** Dr. Jennifer Franz
**Title:** Obstetrician
**Location:** New York

In my experience as an obstetrician, the labor room is where patients are most likely to have an agenda. Patients usually have a labor plan they want to follow, such as avoidance of intervention, IV, fetal monitoring, and so forth. It is my job to follow their wishes as closely as possible as long as I feel their labor plan is medically safe. If I feel that any of those choices might compromise the mothers' health or the health of the fetus then I will discuss the risks of those choices with the patient. This is where all your work in establishing a doctor-patient relationship based on trust pays off and helps to move the two agendas toward alignment.

Every physician-patient relationship is about helping patients reach the right treatment decisions. The basic goal during patient interviews is to obtain information that allows for a diagnosis of the medical situation. I want to establish trust, so my patients feel more comfortable when providing information, especially since evidence-based protocols in my specialty do not always determine the best treatment options. It is important to understand my patients' medical and social-economic needs in order to create the right plan of care. I have found that the most important way to build trust and understanding is to give my patients the time necessary to build this bridge. I never try to rush or coerce a patient into deciding on my recommendations.

Shared decisions should take into account the patient's desired labor experience, such as when to start Pitocin. Obstetricians should also cover choices in labor and delivery that are not absolute medical necessities, such as deciding if the patient should receive an epidural, or when to proceed with an operative vaginal delivery or a C-section. It is important to talk about the protocol during potential emergencies, such as a cord prolapse, so the patient knows ahead of time that shared decisions are not possible should such an emergency arise. This is often a quick conversation based on the emergent situation.

When it comes to labor plans, you have to respect peoples' cultural differences, even if they may not lead to the safest medical choices. This is most common among patients who refuse blood transfusions based on religious beliefs. I try to compromise by tailoring options for treatment based on the risk of bleeding and discussing the possible outcomes. Many of my religious patients also believe birth control is not an acceptable option to them, so if a patient is willing to accept the health risks associated with having additional children, I will review the risks, but ultimately respect their ability to make an informed decision.

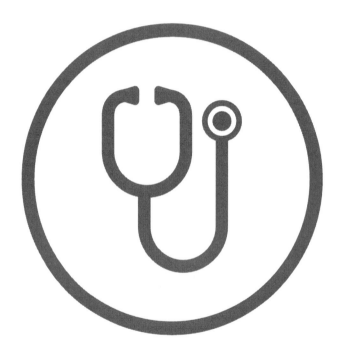

# Chapter 3

# Physician Responses to Patients

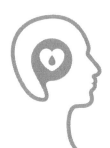

n a 2007 study published in the *Journal of Clinical Oncology*, researchers videotaped conversations between oncologists and their cancer patients to record the number of times the oncologists identified and responded to a major emotion expressed by their patients. Surprisingly, only 22 percent of oncologists in the study capitalized on what researchers referred to as an "empathic opportunity," while 77 percent of the oncologists either ignored the emotion, restated facts, or went on to discuss the management plan. Empathy is a respectful understanding of what others are experiencing. When a patient demonstrates an emotion, an empathic opportunity presents itself as a means of responding in a way that lets the patient know that you understand the experience of receiving serious medical news, and that you will not take their concerns for granted.

As physicians, we can only achieve empathy by forgoing judgment of another person's reactions and using these emotions, however irrational, to serve pragmatic purposes. Researchers in the area of clinical communication often refer to the arousal of emotions in patients as "emotional temperature." For example, researchers would classify a patient in denial as experiencing low emotional temperature while a patient demonstrating anger as experiencing high emotional temperature. When the emotional temperature of a medical interview reaches high intensity, some physicians make the mistake of raising their own emotional temperature in direct proportion to the patient's level of arousal. In Chapter 1, we discussed the dynamics of the doctor-patient relationship and highlighted psychological factors that factor into these types of responses by physicians. Some physicians react poorly if the patient blames them or makes them feel incompetent. Defensive reactions of this nature are self-serving and rarely accomplish anything. The key to dealing with a patient demonstrating high emotional temperature is to act rather than react. A hostile response on the part of the physician is a form of reaction, and you must avoid it at all costs. On the other hand, if you practice professional detachment, the patient will interpret your ability to identify and understand the underlying emotional cause as a lack of interest for their concerns. Instead, you must offer a professional response that mixes professional detachment with empathy. The most common defensive behaviors used by physicians include:

- Asking closed questions as a way to avoid the patient's feelings
- Asking leading questions as a way of indicating blame
- Interrupting the patient's narrative
- Changing a subject that you are not comfortable discussing
- Offering premature assurance as a way to subdue the patient's emotions

- Becoming angry or impatient
- Dismissing psychological symptoms as irrelevant to treatment
- Discussing patients' problems with others without their consent

# Responding to Emotions with Statements

To offer a response that mixes professional detachment with empathy, first check your emotional intensity. If raised, remind yourself that professional detachment is necessary in order to remain objective about the patient's reaction. Next, ask yourself, "How would I feel if I were in this patient's situation?" Imagining your own reaction allows you to appreciate what the patient feels, even if your reaction to the same situation might be different. Before you respond to a high-intensity situation, you must first interpret the response and determine if it is normal for the situation, or pathological. Interpretation of the emotional reaction requires three steps:

## Step 1

**Identify the emotion.** (You think, "This patient is expressing anger.")

## Step 2

**Identify the cause of the emotion.** (You think, "This patient is experiencing physical pain and is expressing anger as a symptom of the pain.")

## Step 3

**Show the patient that you have made a connection between the emotion and its cause.** (You say, "I can appreciate how angry you must be at the physical pain you are experiencing.")

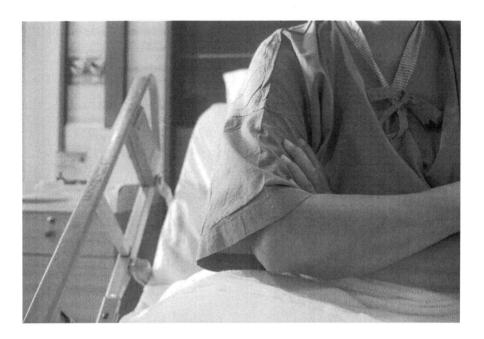

# Empathic Statements

The empathic response is the most effective way to respond to a patient's emotions. As the physician, you do not have to experience the emotion yourself (i.e. sympathy); the key is to demonstrate a form of support. As exampled by Step 3, an empathic statement is a form of emotional restatement, whereby you verbally name the emotion and the source. In the example provided, "I can appreciate" is the empathic statement, "angry" identifies the emotion and "physical pain" names the source. As a rule of thumb, you should always directly address high-temperature reactions with empathy, and handle low-temperature reactions with more subtlety. Denial, as an example, requires an indirect approach since the unconscious is driving the emotional reaction. In either case, the physician must acknowledge and address the temperature regardless of intensity, or further communication cannot continue.

Using the empathic response not only acknowledges the emotion, but also allows the patient to elaborate further. In Chapter 2, we discussed the use of the E4 model as a way of distinguishing between what the *body* is experiencing and what the *person* is experiencing. The empathic statement, therefore, is the process task that further elicits the patient's story as a means of creating that distinction. However, only use empathic statements if you are certain of the emotion and cause, as incorrectly naming an emotion and cause may cause the patient resentment. If the emotion remains uncertain to you, proceed to responding with an open question (discussed later in this chapter).

## Factual Statements

In some cases, giving direct, factual information is the best response. This is especially true when the physician has named despair as the emotion and the cause of despair indicates that the patient is looking for hope. According to the *Handbook of Communication in Oncology and Palliative Care*, "Current guidelines recommend that [physicians] balance honest disclosure with sustaining hope… Clinicians can begin by exploring sources of hope, identifying potential obstacles, and shifting to affirming personal attributes and qualities that convey the value of the person." As in the case of the empathic statement, the danger of providing factual statements rests in the potential of naming the emotion too early. In this case, you risk appearing professionally detached by providing information the patient neither wanted nor requested. Before you provide the patient with any facts, consider negotiating the amount of disclosure you would consider helpful while concurrently sustaining hope. You might lead with, "It sounds like you want me to discuss the facts of the illness." If the patient wants information but needs to remain hopeful, you may begin negotiating the amount of disclosure by saying, "Help me understand your preferences for the level of detail you like in the information I will give you." To determine how much content provides enough facts and retains hope, use your clinical knowledge and experience to estimate the risks and benefits of the information.

At some point in your career, you probably have encountered patients awaiting test results, and they asked for the facts as soon as you walked into the room. When patients anxiously demand the facts, identify the emotional anxiety, then acknowledge the anxiety with an empathic preparatory statement like, "I realize you are worried about the test results, so we are going to use this time to talk about the results and what that means for your immediate future." An empathic statement like that acknowledges the emotion, allows you time to create a soothing environment, prepares the patient for the facts, and helps the patient refocus on the agenda and away from the anxiety.

## Aggressive Statements

Hostility is one of the most detrimental counter-responses a physician can give to a patient expressing blind emotion. While you have the freedom in your personal life to respond combatively against someone exhibiting the same behavior, it is unprofessional to launch a counterattack against your patient for the sake of defending yourself. While an aggressive response may get the patient to squelch their emotion or act according to your clinical agenda, the long-term consequences to the clinical relationship are greater than the short-term gains. An aggressive response lacks empathy, mirrors the patient's emotional temperature, and often places blame at the feet of the patient. An aggressive response also takes the form of a judgmental response. Consider the following aggressive/judgmental responses toward a patient with high emotional temperature:

>**Patient:** "You told me this disease had a chance of being cured. If you don't know what you're talking about, then I'm getting a second opinion."

>**Doctor:** "Fine, go ahead and get a second opinion. The next doctor is going to tell you the same thing. You only have yourself to blame for this problem anyway."

In all likelihood, neither you nor most of your colleagues would ever consider responding to a patient this way, but in all probability, you know someone with a reputation for using aggressive statements or passive-aggression as a form of clinical dialogue. Without even knowing it, they wear the label as the doctor without any "bedside manner." Physicians who lack bedside manner often lack an understanding for the distinction between professional and social contracts. Professional contracts contain implicit agreements between two parties that are more limiting than the contracts of ordinary social interactions. In other words, the actions that society allows you take in daily life are prohibitive in the professional world. Under a professional contract, the physician agrees to use his or her expertise to the benefit of the patient rather than to gain advantage or exploit the patient's vulnerability. While no legal obligation exists, 98 percent of American medical students and 50 percent of British medical students have sworn some form of oath. If you or your colleagues respond to your patients with aggressive or judgmental statements, you are violating that oath. To that end, the Declaration of Geneva, published by the World Medical Association, reads:

- I will practice my profession with conscience and dignity;
- I will not use my medical knowledge to violate human rights and civil liberties, even under threat.

## Reassuring Statements

Some physicians make the mistake of considering reassurance as a form of empathy. When a patient is looking for hope, the physician might offer a reassuring response out of a natural instinct to provide hope. The reassuring response tells the patient, "Do not worry; you will be fine." Though intended as a form of comfort, if the physician uses the reassuring response too early (before they have heard the patient's concerns), the patient may misinterpret this offering as a lazy means of emotional support and create the opposite effect. The key to ensuring a proper reassuring response is to give one after you have heard the patient's concerns, not before.

If you use the reassuring response at all, remember to balance hope with honest disclosure. Without some form of balance, you not only risk inflating expectations that may go unmet by treatment, but also misinterpretation if you do not check the patient for understanding of your reassuring response. For example, if you use euphemisms to soften the blow of bad news, you may wind up confusing the patient about their prognosis. In cases of cancer recurrence where doctors work to provide reassurance or soften the blow through euphemisms, you often will hear the patient say something like, "But I thought you said I had nothing to worry about." Even if the doctor never said this, the patient hears something entirely different when communication lacks precision. Such cases leave doctors looking blameworthy and having to explain things they cannot answer.

# Responding to Emotions with Questions

The use of statements and continuers signal the patient to continue talking about their condition. Likewise, the physician can elicit the patient's story by asking questions. Two kinds of questions exist for this purpose: open and closed. Open questions, by their nature, prevent patients from giving limited "yes" or "no" responses and give the patient leeway to talk at length, expressing as much detail as they want. When the patient expresses an emotion, you have two options. You can use an empathic statement to acknowledge emotion or use an open question to explore the meaning of the emotion. Open questions serve as investigative tools when you are probing for answers and discover a new angle to the patient's story. The open question will lead to responses that help you determine whether to continue pursuing a theory about what is happening to the person or the body. In some cases, the patient will express the need for facts through a buried question. A buried question is a question not overtly expressed as a question, but rather a statement. In this instance, you would use an open statement to confirm if you need to use a factual statement to deliver information the patient needs. Consider the following example of a statement expressed as a buried question, followed by the physician probing the statement with an open question.

> **Patient:** "My mother's doctor diagnosed her last week with hemochromatosis. He says it is an autosomal recessive disorder, which means that a child must inherit a mutant gene from both parents in order to get it."

> **Doctor:** "What did you hope to find out by seeing me?"

The subtext buried the patient's statement would seem to indicate that the patient has questions about the possibility of genetic inheritance and the likelihood of contracting the same disease. The buried question may also hint toward an underlying emotion: concern, fear, anxiety, and so forth. Following the buried question with an open question enables the physician to confirm the existence of the buried question and name the emotion and its cause. As a rule of thumb, it is safer to use the open question before the empathic statement because it reduces the risk of making the wrong assumption about the patient's feelings. The open question creates certainty about the emotion and its cause by eliciting the patient narrative; the empathic response acknowledges the emotion and its cause once you have narrowed it down. Always start with the open question if you are uncertain. Some typical questions designed to prompt the patient narrative include:

- Can you tell me what you are thinking?
- Can you help me understand what has been happening?
- Can you tell me what went wrong?
- What do you think caused the problem?
- Can you tell me when this started happening?

Closed questions focus on limited "yes," "no," or multiple choice answers; they work best for when you have narrowed down a theory and your focus is confirming your theory. For example, if the patient begins a narrative based on an open question, and the narrative reveals symptoms of a disorder you can readily identify, you then would employ closed questions to confirm the disorder as a possible diagnosis. As a rule, you should always avoid using a closed question after a patient has expressed an emotion. Consider the following example of an emotion expressed by the patient followed by a closed question, framed empathically:

> **Patient:** "I've been experiencing shortness of breath and numbness in my arms, but I think it's because I've been feeling

anxious and under a lot of stress lately. I just found out that my mother has a heart condition."

**Doctor:** "Are you afraid that heart disease runs in the family?"

Is the emotion controlling the stress really anxiety, or is it something else, like anger? If the emotion is anger, is the anger originating from the patient's anxiety about their individual health, or anxiety about the mother's health? We have no way of knowing if we elicit limited responses through closed questioning. In this example, the patient expresses an apparent emotion (anxiety) and the doctor rushes to an assumption by naming the emotion and its cause without confirming it. As a closed question, the physician is also likely to get limited information from a limited response, not to mention that it risks making the patient feel unheard if the assumption proves incorrect.

# Distinguishing Patient Behaviors

After determining an emotion and its causes, you will have to decide whether the emotion the patient exhibits is adaptive or maladaptive to the cycle of grief process. Given the nature of bad news, what may seem like abnormal behavior may be normal under circumstances that involve receiving serious, life-changing news. Behaviors that help the patient cope with or recover from their illness are adaptive traits that physicians should encourage. Behaviors detrimental to the clinical agenda and destructive to the patient's well-being are maladaptive. Sometimes, distinguishing between adaptive and maladaptive behavior takes time and requires lengthy observation. Denial, for example, can be an adaptive behavior as an initial coping mechanism, but if it lingers for too long, denial may become a destructive force to treatment goals. Simply put, the patients who do not believe they are sick may refuse to discuss a treatment regimen. As previously discussed in Chapter 1, patients sometimes linger for too long around one stage of the grief cycle and require support from the physician in order to move forward into the next stage. In rare cases, the patient may not need to reach the acceptance stage if the behavior appears supportive to the patient's needs and the clinical agenda.

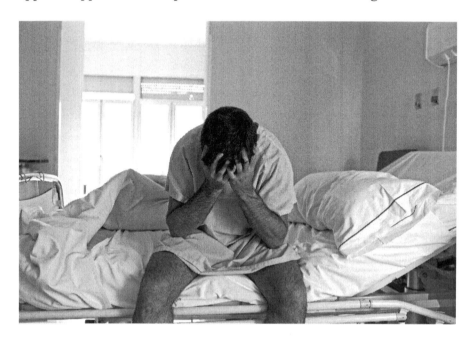

## *Denial as Adaptive or Maladaptive*

Denial is a cognitive defense mechanism that protects a person against anxiety created by life-altering news. When denial appears on the grief cycle, common symptoms may include behavior that appears too normal for the circumstances, illogical behavior, non-compliance, and non-integration of medical information into the patient's personal world. While the symptoms of denial can help you identify the behaviors as belonging to denial, you must also measure the emotional temperature of denial. From lowest to highest intensity, the spectrum of denial begins with mild forms of forgetting, such as forgetting what the doctor said, forgetting about medication, or forgetting about the seriousness of diagnosis. The patient also may procrastinate when it comes to following the physician's directions, like picking up medication or scheduling another doctor visit. Denial becomes more serious if the patient begins to minimize the gravity of the situation or shows signs of conscious suppression. Subconsciously, disavowal of the situation is the most intense form of denial on the spectrum, and the most frequently maladaptive. In other words, if the patient suppresses the memory of the interview or the perception of their health, they will see your treatment plan as illogical and preposterous. The longer the patient experiences subconscious disavowal, the more likely the symptoms will play a destructive role in the patient's needs and clinical agenda.

The key variables to consider when determining the intensity of denial are the degree to which the patient expresses denial and the degree to which their need to cope interferes with facing the actual threat. If the symptoms of denial appear on the low end of the spectrum and do not impair their ability to make proper treatment decisions, then denial as a defense mechanism is adaptive. If denial appears on the high end of the spectrum and presents itself as a form of psychosis, which impedes memory, perception, treatment goals, and the patient's needs, then denial as a defense mechanism is maladaptive. The level of intensity also may fluctuate between high and low depending on how the patient's perception of the threat changes over time.

One might argue that if denial is a form of self-protection, and the patient uses denial to alleviate distress, then would not denial serve the patient's needs while impeding the clinical agenda? It is certainly possible, but if the clinical agenda means the difference between life and death, then the patient is adversely using denial as a form of self-protection. In this scenario, the patient is putting their life at risk by decreasing their distress. In some cases, upon the family's wishes, you might be inclined to support the patient's behavior by denying the patient information. However, your ethical responsibility as a health care professional is to determine when denial is beneficial before you accept this type of complicity. So how do you determine when denial is beneficial? One way is to predict how behaviors associated with denial might have a positive impact on the disease trajectory. According to the *Handbook of Communication in Oncology and Palliative Care*, a 15-year prospective study of adjustment styles in breast cancer patients showed that "women who used a fighting spirit or denial as coping strategies survived longer than those who reacted with stoic acceptance or helplessness." When denial correlates with hope, the behavior is more likely to be adaptive. If denial expressed as hope interferes with the patient realizing death as an eventuality, then the patient's behavior is maladaptive to preparations for death (such as making out a will) and may add distress to the bereaved. In order to address denial you must:

### Step 1

Recognize the behavior as symptoms of denial and employ the process task of finding out how much the patient knows, asking open questions like, "Could you tell me what you know about the problem?"

### Step 2

Determine if the symptoms are adaptive or maladaptive by employing the process tasks. This involves determining the patient's past reactions to stress and the behavior's impact on the clinical agenda through questioning (ex: How have you coped with difficult situations in the past? / How are you managing at home or at work?).

## Step 3

Determine if the denial requires management.

## Step 4

Explore the psychological causes of the denial by asking open questions about coping. Acknowledge the emotional reaction with an empathic statement like, "It's normal to experience difficulty in coping, but sometimes if we explore the emotions surrounding that difficulty, it becomes easier to deal with them."

## Step 5

Provide factual statements that merge the patient's needs with the goals of care. Process tasks include clarifying the patient's prefer-ence on information, decision-making, and goals of care.

## Step 6

Be aware of cultural issues in relation to denial. Process tasks may include using an interpreter or asking family members to educate you regarding their cultural norms for clinical encounters.

## Step 7

Monitor the fluctuation of denial along the illness trajectory and reassess its status as adaptive or maladaptive. If it gradually becomes clear that the behavior is becoming maladaptive, use the process task of asking the patient to explain their status and phase of treatment. Use sensitivity and tact by asking questions like, "Does the fact that your condition has worsened over the last two months make you think it may be something more serious?" Following your discussions, determine if denial's level of intensity has lowered or increased.

## Step 8

Support the patient by scheduling follow-up visits.

# The NURSE Protocol

Given how long it takes to determine whether a behavior is adaptive or maladaptive, we can begin to understand why tracking emotion is so important. Because emotions may fluctuate between clinical interviews and during the course of the illness trajectory, you always have to know the patient's current state of readiness for the next consultation, the next test, or the next medical treatment. Whenever you attempt to name the patient's emotion, the NURSE protocol can help you avoid overstating the emotion in an unskilled way that labels the patient.

Similar to the theoretical models of communication, the NURSE protocol forms an acronym. This protocol reiterates the process tasks covered in this chapter, but with a wrinkle — once you have named and understood the emotion, encourage adaptive behavior by praising the patient's efforts, however small they may seem. Promote this subtle form of encouragement by reminding the patient that you and your staff will not abandon them. Completing these two steps with skill sets the table for exploring the emotion and turning detrimental behavior toward positive progress. For example, you can avoid overstating an emotion and labeling a person's behavior by framing your responses with verbal qualifiers such as, "It sounds like," or "It must be hard to…" The use of such framing techniques let the patient know you are making a guess and trying to understand what is going on.

**N**ame the emotion

**U**nderstand the emotion

**R**espect and praise the patient

**S**upport the patient

**E**xplore the emotion

## Additional Listening Techniques

When the emotional temperature is high, letting the patient know that you have heard their concerns plays an integral part of support. There are three ways to let the patient know you have heard their concerns: repetition, reiteration, and reflection. In Chapter 2, we discussed the technique of listening to the patient's vocabulary to determine the level of "med-speak" you can use to discuss the medical problem. The technique of repetition works in similar fashion. You listen to the patient's words, keying in on emotional buzzwords to explore, and then leading your next response with one or two buzzwords from the patient's last sentence. For example, if the patient cites dizziness as a side effect of the medicine they have been taking, you would repeat the buzzword "dizzy" by saying, "So the medicine has been making you dizzy?" Notice the response is a rhetorical question rather than a closed question. Rhetorical questions restate what the listener has heard; closed questions would elicit a limited "yes", "no," or multiple choice response. Leading with a rhetorical question that repeats the buzzword from the patient's last sentence lets the patient know you have listened and that you still control the dialogue. This verbal cue gives you the option of eliciting the patient narrative with any of the responses covered in this chapter. If your goal is to demonstrate listening but also direct the patient narrative in a subtle but certain direction, you may use the technique of reiteration. Reiteration repeats the buzzwords used by the patient, but repeats them in your own words if you suspect your description might be more appropriate. Reflection takes this idea further and interprets the entire narrative rather than one or two buzzwords. To reflect upon the patient's narrative, you might lead with, "So if I understand what you are saying correctly…" Reflection as a listening technique allows the patient to confirm your understanding as correct or provides them the opportunity to clarify their own narrative.

# Responding to Anger

While anger can be a symptom of pain, several different emotions, such as fear and guilt, can manifest as anger. In your exploration of the patient's emotions, you may discover that the underlying emotion of a patient reacting with anger may be the impending fear of losing control or physical attractiveness. Some underlying causes of anger may appear more abstract than other underlying causes — for example, anger toward a disease that may take away their control, their life aspirations, chances of life fulfillment, and the perception that these negative possibilities are of random chance. Sometimes patients direct their anger toward a specific object or person, namely themselves, their family, the doctors, or social institutions. When confronted by patients who demonstrate anger toward specific or abstract causes, consider how you want to redirect the patient's behavior using the responses outlined in this chapter, their intended outcomes, and choose the best course of action. For example, if a patient tells you that they are going to sue the previous doctor, you could respond with an open question, closed question, an empathic statement, a factual statement, an aggressive statement, or show that you have listened through a repetitive, reiterative, or reflective statement. When choosing your response, ask yourself, "How will the patient react to each response, and will this response direct the patient toward the goals I want to set?" In other words, you must anticipate which outcome each response will likely provoke. For example:

The patient says, "The doctor made the wrong diagnosis and my condition got worse! I considered giving that idiot a one-star review on Yelp™."

**1**   **You respond with a closed question:** "Did your previous doctor order a test?"

**The potential outcome:** The patient provides some limited facts, but the narrative is likely to be short and even less likely to determine whether the previous doctor was at fault.

**2**   **You respond with an open question:** "Why do you feel he was to blame?"

**The potential outcome:** Avoids participation in blaming another professional and redirects the narrative on exploration of the patient's anger.

**3**   **You respond with an empathic statement:** "You sound angry that the condition turned out to be something else."

**The potential outcome:** You elicit the emotional narrative to determine the real source of the anger. The response raises the emotional temperature, but remains a calculated risk because the patient is directing the anger at someone else.

**You respond with a factual statement:** "These symptoms are present in a wide range of diseases, so the diagnostic accuracy rate tends to be a little lower."

**The potential outcome:** You inform the patient but reduce the patient's hope that an accurate diagnosis can immediately be determined.

**You respond with a reassuring statement:** "I'm sure you were right about the doctor. We'll get it right this time."

**The potential outcome:** You blame another professional without enough information. You offer the patient hope, but run the risk of giving the patient false hope and having the patient blame you too if your diagnosis proves incorrect.

**You respond with an aggressive statement:** "You expect doctors to get things right every time? You need to learn how to be more patient."

**The potential outcome:** You destroy the clinical relationship, and the patient loses trust in you and/or becomes uncooperative for the remainder of the relationship.

**You find the buzzwords and respond with a repetitive, reiterative, or reflective statement:** "It sounds like you are angry that the wrong diagnosis has wasted valuable time and might lead to a condition that eventually becomes very threatening."

**The potential outcome:** The patient feels heard but expects you to continue talking.

# The Nine-Step Approach to Anger

Unfortunately, there is a measure of self-sacrifice in being open to receiving complaints, as statistical evidence shows that doctors who receive complaints are more likely to feel professionally assaulted and more likely to change their rapport with the patient. In a study published in the *New Zealand Medical Journal*, author Wayne Cunningham revealed that, "The doctor's emotional state, their attitude towards their work and patients, and their ability to cope with the stresses of practice may all impact on their ability to deliver high quality care." Cunningham also noted that, "American literature suggests that a complaint represents an assault on the recipient doctor's sense of self and personal integrity. Canadian literature indicates that complaints can cause an increase in both positive and negative defensive medicine, and British and European literature suggests that complaints cause changes in doctor's behaviors that are predicated by concern for the doctor-patient relationship."

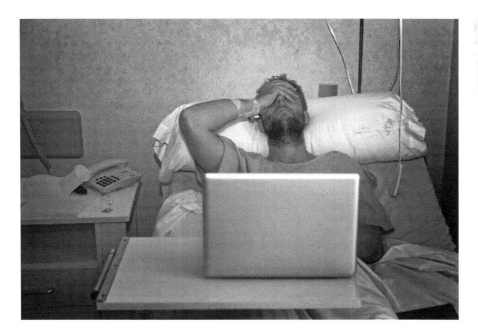

In short, complaints should lead to improved medical practice, but the study conducted by Cunningham indicates that "some of that study's [physicians] held persisting emotional responses (such as depression or anger), some had an altered perception of themselves as doctors, and some indicated an erosion of goodwill towards patients. The implication of that study was that complaints might reduce (rather than improve) the delivery of patient care." Sometimes the only way to help the patient is to receive the brunt of their anger, and the only way you can do so constructively is to control your emotional state. You can find techniques for reducing distress at **www.mentalhealth.com/mag1/p51-str.html**. For doctors ready and willing to face their patients' wrath, the *Handbook of Communication in Oncology and Palliative Care* offers a nine-step approach in responding to anger. The purpose of this approach is to shift the patient's perspective from anger and distress to something less distressful and more constructive.

## Step 1: Preparation

If a patient is angry, try to coordinate with nurses or other colleagues by informing the next-in-line practitioner about the patient's emotional state and temperature. Grapevine information should include the causes of the anger (if known), the object of the anger (a person or thing), and recommendations for reducing the patient's distress (such as moving the interview setting to a quiet conference room where everyone can sit).

## Step 2: Listen

Use the listening techniques discussed in this chapter to encourage a mutual understanding of the situation after the patient has vented and aired grievances. The communication goals set here should achieve an understanding by the physician of the problem as the patient sees it, and an examination of any differing perceptions that exist between the patient and physician.

## Step 3: Offer empathic acknowledgement

Use the empathic statement to allow the patient to air his or her grievances. Think of this process as a psychotherapeutic strategy in which the focus is not on your medical integrity, but the patient's well-being.

## Step 4: Provide symptom relief

While listening to the complaint, look for the symptoms that are causing the anger. Sometimes patients become angry for a simple reason: They are in pain. If the complaint reveals the underlying symptom causing the anger, your communication goal in responding to the anger should be relief of the symptom(s) causing it.

## Step 5: Involve experienced professionals

If the anger persists, and you have concluded (by taking their personal history) that the patient's anger fits a lifelong pattern of behavior, you may need to involve a psychotherapist or social worker. If you decide to bring in professionals, be sure to coordinate your efforts with these professionals, include the junior staff, and make sure everyone universally agrees on the goals of care.

## Step 6: Reconsider your approach

This step is an outgrowth of Step 5. When the anger persists, consider calling a meeting with the staff to brainstorm a new approach and eliminate confusion.

## Step 7: Consider setting limits

If anger becomes extreme to the point that the medical staff may be subject to physical danger, consider limiting interactions with the patient. In these cases, you may have to arrange a conjunctive meeting to discuss these interactions with your senior staff and the patient's family.

## Step 8: Support the medical team

Develop a detailed care plan that involves all team members, especially if outside professionals are included.

## Step 9: Involve an independent broker

Offer to get the patient a second opinion from an independent health professional. The independent broker acts as a mediator and offers judgment or proposes remedy of the situation. The independent broker may help both parties reach an agreement that reduces the patient's anger. However, be aware that if you decide to use an independent broker and the broker rules in your favor, this may cause the patient to feel invalidated and further exacerbate the anger. Therefore, if you go to an independent broker, you will need assurance that if the broker agrees with your perspective, he or she will present the ruling tactfully and offer a compromise designed to reduce the patient's distress.

# Identifying Prolonged Distress

Prolonged distress is synonymous with suffering. However, suffering is not always synonymous with physical pain. When suffering does not manifest itself physically, you must explore the nature of psychological suffering. To assist a person who is suffering, your focus should be on reintegrating the patient toward involvement in the world while steering them away from the type of demoralization that causes all forms of withdrawal. For dealing with anger in a palliative care setting, see Appendix F. Some useful solicitations for the patient's suffering narrative may include the following phrases:

- When was the last time you were feeling good?
- Describe what made you decide to go to the doctor.
- If you are suffering, tell me exactly what you are feeling.

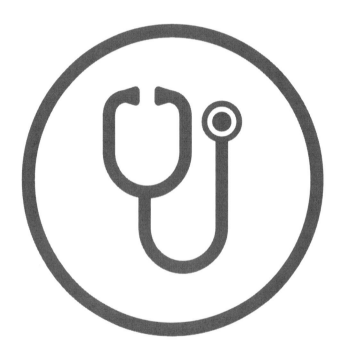

# Chapter 4

# How to Discuss Prognosis

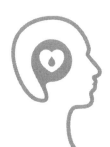

ow we present negative medical news in a positive light not only relates to how we disclose what we already know about a patient's health situation, but also relates to how we provide an estimate of the illness trajectory. When patients need hope and want reassurance, they ask about prognosis. Prognosis in the context of health care involves different elements of medical forecasting, which vary in degree of concern to the patient. The challenge is determining which elements of prognosis the patient wants, and how much information they want disclosed. The elements of prognosis may include:

- The chances of a specific health state occurring or recurring
- The degree of physical or mental impairment

- The expected symptoms
- The expected benefits of therapy
- The expected side effects of therapy
- The likelihood of survival
- The amount of time the patient has left to live

No universal guideline exists for determining which elements of prognosis patients want their doctors to give them. When it comes to getting a prognosis, studies in palliative and hospice care indicate a wide range of patient preferences. In a 2007 study published in *Journal of Pain and Symptom Management*, results showed that "physicians tended to underestimate the information needs of patients… as many physicians believed they had provided the patient with more information than the patient perceived to be the case. Even when physicians believed they had given the patient information, a subgroup of patients did not understand their diagnosis and treatment." The study also revealed "a consistent discrepancy between patient and physician reports as to the extent of the disease and the aims of treatments, as well as the level of information." These studies not only intimate the level of difficulty in communicating prognosis, but also the subsequent problems that arise when physicians inaccurately judge the patient's views and preferences by taking a universal approach to prognosis. Therefore, as a physician, you will need to assess your patients' prognosis needs on a case-by-case basis using the skills outlined in this chapter.

# The Psychology of Doctor and Patient Expectations

In Chapter 1, we discussed how emotional and psychological factors of bad news influence the behaviors of both patients and physicians. Because physicians experience a range of emotions when it comes to delivering bad news (fears of being sued for malpractice, causing the patient distress, or disappointing the patient's expectations), they tend to offer premature reassurance or shy away from giving a diagnosis altogether. Life-threatening illnesses typically trigger three questions from patients that cause doctors to give premature reassurance or avoid prognosis. They include:

- How long do I have to live?
- Is my condition fatal?
- What problems am I going to experience in this process?

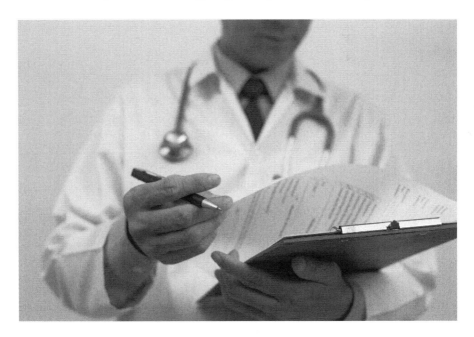

As the saying goes, the more you know, the less you understand. Doctors dislike answering these types of questions because their experience has likely taught them that prognostication of an individual illness is inexact and providing concrete answers only invites the possibility of looking incompetent for being wrong. Palliative care specialists forced to prognosticate an illness trajectory run the risk of admitting another failure if their prognosis proves incorrect — the failure of their treatment plan to generate the expected outcome. Premature reassurance comes into play when the physician fears that giving a bleak prognosis might prompt the patient to seek a second opinion, which the physician may view as a vote of no confidence in their ability to prognosticate.

Prognostication also tangles with misperception when physicians incorrectly process what the patient is asking. For example, if the patient asks if the illness is terminal, but you interpret this question as a need to know how long he or she has to live, your prognosis will cause the patient to experience shock over the unexpected answer. In short, prognostication based on misinterpreted questions increases the likelihood of disappointing the patient's expectations. Unintended consequences of prognosis can occur even when the patient has greatly diminished expectations. If the patient already knows they are dying, they likely want a prognosis that gives them an idea of what to expect out of the dying process. If your prognosis leaves the patient unprepared for the actual symptoms, you risk raising the emotional temperature directed toward you when the symptoms occur, and thus the amount of distress endured by both parties.

So what exactly do patients want? The answer is to take a patient-centered approach. Since most patients experience conflict between what they fear hearing and what they want to know, it is generally accepted practice to ask patients if they want prognostic information before disclosing it. Although physicians should treat prognosis on a case-by-case basis, statistical evidence shows that patients have strong opinions on how physicians should deliver prognosis. In a mail survey conducted by Stan A. Kaplowitz, results found that 80 percent of patients with either curable or incurable cancer wanted a qualitative prognosis (i.e. Am I terminal?), 50 percent wanted a quantitative estimate (i.e. What is the survival rate?), and overall, those with poorer prognoses were less likely to request prognostic information. In another study conducted by Rebecca Hagerty, only 59 percent of responding patients wanted to know how long they had to live after diagnosis. Eleven percent of patients preferred never to discuss dying and palliative care, and 21 percent indicated that they only wanted the information if they asked directly. Studies of terminally ill patients suggest that while many patients may prefer delaying disclosure or not knowing their prognosis at all, an assessment of patients' current desires may change over time, and therefore the physician may need to renegotiate preferences in diagnostic disclosure at various points along the illness trajectory.

# Communication Challenges on an Illness Trajectory

When patients are encouraged to ask questions, prognosis is the one area where doctors will receive the most questions. If you are the primary care physician for patients with a serious, ongoing illness, you will probably have to discuss and reappraise prognosis at various points along the illness trajectory as it unfolds. The discussion of prognosis is the area of managed care that will present the most communication challenges. Mapping out your patients' probable needs and their interactions with health professionals will help you anticipate any communication challenges you may encounter along the way. While individual diseases run along their own unique trajectories, consider using a universal illness trajectory pattern as a theoretical model for anticipating the service needs of chronic illness. For example, Joanne Lynn and David M. Adamson produced a 2003 RAND Corporation white paper (illustrated in the figure below), which conceptualized patient function in three illness trajectory models of chronic illness. These three models classify people who are sick enough to die into three types: short period of decline, long-term limitations, and prolonged dwindling. Each model uses the trajectory of decline over time that is characteristic of each major type of disease or disability.

*Figure 5. Chronic Illness Trajectory #1*

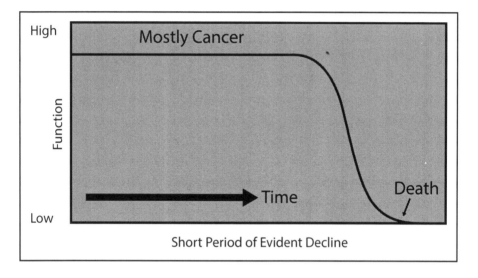

Some illnesses allow the patient to maintain comfort and functioning for a substantial period, followed by a short and rapid decline. Patients with cancer are most likely to function on this type of illness trajectory. If the illness becomes overwhelming, the patient's status usually declines rapidly in the final weeks and days preceding death. Hospice is an important part of the care for this trajectory. When prognosis takes a turn for the worst, the communication challenge on this illness trajectory includes knowing how to discuss the prognosis, which informs the patient of the likely path of the trajectory, and how to discuss transition to hospice care. When patients maintaining comfort and functioning learn that their decline will be sudden and rapid, the emotional shock may prevent them from hearing the prognosis. Therefore, when first- and second-line treatments fail, your communication challenge is to check the patient's understanding and provide prognosis about the likely success of treatment going forward without destroying hope. When death is imminent, the most daunting communication challenge doctors face is the discussion about ending treatment and DNR orders. In some cases, if the illness trajectory brings on sudden, unexpected death, your communication challenge resides in handling the strong emotions of the family who may feel taken by surprise. In other cases, you may have to offer a prognosis when it comes to forecasting the probability of a healthy patient developing an illness for which they have yet to show any symptoms. For example, if a genetic test reveals a faulty BRCA1 gene, and you calculate an 83 percent risk of the patient contracting breast cancer, your communication challenge is to execute the protocols for disclosure for this highly specialized discussion. For protocols on genetic testing disclosure, contact your local or national medical association.

*Figure 6. Chronic Illness Trajectory #2*

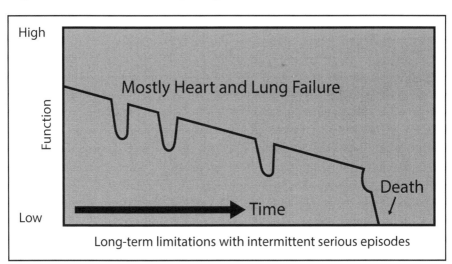

If you prognosticate an illness in which you expect the patient to live for a relatively long time with minor limitations in everyday life, the illness may follow trajectory #2 and present periodic physiological stresses that lead to a worsening of serious symptoms. For example, patients with heart and lung diseases commonly fit into this trajectory and may die from a sudden complication or exacerbation of symptoms, such as bodily stresses resulting from inflammation in the lungs. Your communication challenge on this trajectory would include prognostication of potential complications, as well as the discussion of advance-care planning in relation to the prognosis. You also may need to have a do-not resuscitate (DNR) discussion about discontinuing ventilation should the patient wind up in ICU following an unexpected complication. DNR orders typically require input from the executors, so the physician's communication challenge might also involve getting the patient's permission to hold a family meeting to educate them as to the prognosis, the potential complications on the illness trajectory, and their role in a possible DNR scenario. Unexpected death on this trajectory is also common due to the unpredictable nature of complications associated with long-term illness.

*Figure 7. Chronic Illness Trajectory #3*

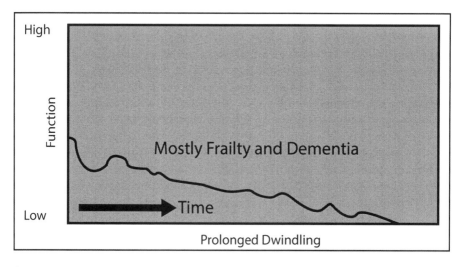

Prolonged illnesses tend to result from battles with previous illness and therefore functioning at the beginning of this trajectory is likely to start low. Patients who survive illnesses like cancer or chronic obstructive pulmonary disease are likely to die at older ages of either neurological failure (such as Alzheimer's or other dementia) or generalized frailty of multiple body systems. Your communication challenges along this illness trajectory may include prognosis about disease recurrence to avoid demoralization or discussions about unexpected or severe side effects from the disease. When side effects diminish the patient's quality of life, they may feel cheated when their disease has departed but left them with disabilities.

Though all three of these theoretical models represent patients who face life-threatening problems, they demonstrate statistical reliability and can be a useful starting point for tailoring health services to the individual's needs. According to Lynn and Adamson, "Analyses of Medicare claims show that about one-fifth of those who die have a course consistent with [illness trajectory #1]; another fifth share the course of [illness trajectory #2]; and two-fifths follow [illness trajectory #3]. The last one-fifth split between those who die suddenly and others we have not yet learned to classify."

# Negotiating Disclosure about Illness

Although a prognostic interview may occur after you have interviewed the patient about his or her initial diagnosis, the rules of engagement are relatively the same. Before discussing diagnosis, ensure that the discussion takes place in privacy, free of interruptions, and ask if the patient would like others present. Once you have initiated the session and gathered information about what the patient knows, the next step in the prognostic interview is negotiating the agenda. Negotiating the agenda involves two steps.

**Step 1**

Asking if the patient wants information about prognosis.

**Step 2**

Exploring with the patient preferences as to the type of information they want, and in what format.

Step 1 requires that you frame the question by saying something like, "If you want, I can tell you what happens to most people in your situation. Would you like me to talk about your prognosis?" You might follow this by saying that you cannot predict the patient's illness trajectory or response to treatment with complete certainty, although describing what you have seen in other cases should give the patient an idea about possible outcomes. However, you should also preface any statement on statistical prognostic estimates with a statement about the limitations of prognostic formulations, especially if these limitations give the patient a modicum of hope. If the patient agrees to hear the prognosis, proceed to telling the patient that you would like to explore their information preferences. You might follow this listing the most common elements of prognosis (or those most relevant to the illness), explaining what each prognostic element means, asking the patient which elements he or she would like to discuss, and in what type of format the patient would like the elements presented. The most common elements to negotiate in a prognostic agenda include:

- Staging details (evaluation of the extent of disease)
- Format desired (e.g. words, numbers or graphs)
- Chance of cure
- Chance of remission

- Chance of recurrence
- Possible short-term side effects of treatment recommendations
- Possible long-term side effects of treatment recommendations
- Survival estimates

As you explain your way through the list of prognostic elements, make sure you are able to provide the most current information and cite the source. If you offer information that you believe may change as studies reveal new insights, be prepared to give the patient an estimate on when new prognostic information may become available. Your estimate should involve a range (i.e. "six-to-12 months") as opposed to an approximation (i.e. "about 12 months"). According to a 2004 study of diagnostic discussion preferences published in the *Journal of Clinical Oncology*, patients preferred words and numbers rather than pie charts or graphs as a format for diagnostic discussion. Patients in this study reported that the use of words and numbers seemed more optimistic and hopeful whereas pie charts and graphs felt too clinical, dogmatic, and unspecific to the individual illness. The same study also reported that patients with metastatic disease expecting to survive for years were more likely to want to discuss how long they might live than those who expected to live only a few weeks or months. Therefore, if your prognostication matches the patient's initial life expectancy, your patient is more likely to want more disclosure than a patient whose initial life expectancy does not match your prognostication.

Once you begin to talk about treatments, divide the conversation into an explanation of potential risks if the patient chooses treatment and potential risks if the patient chooses to go without treatment. If you offer risk reduction possibilities, provide examples of your calculations. Once you have outlined the potential risks and benefits of treatment, your conversation should branch out into the disease's potential impact on the patient's lifestyle. While talking about the personal impact on day-to-day living, emphasize the hope-giving aspects of information without giving premature reassurance. Check the patient for understanding at various points, and pause to allow the patient an opportunity to renegotiate his or her information preferences. As you move the interview to a close, check the patient for understanding by summarizing the main points of the consultation, re-emphasize the hope-giving aspects, offer referral support, and indicate your availability for future consultations.

How you negotiate prognostic disclosure with the patient may differ from how you frame the prognosis. Doctors faced with the challenge of forecasting negative or potentially life-threatening news fall into one of three categories: realists, optimists, and avoiders. Realistic doctors emphasize respect for patient autonomy. They believe that in order to make informed decisions, the patient must have the appropriate amount of prognostic information necessary to make informed decisions about their future. Though realists support informed behavior, they risk appearing too blunt and uncaring in their methods of communication. Optimists emphasize support for the patient's hopes; they believe that positive reinforcement can aid recovery. Statistically, this is not an altogether unrealistic approach.

When denial correlates with hope, the behavior is more likely to be adaptive, as you may recall an earlier study mentioned in Chapter 1 that showed longer survival rates in breast cancer patients who used optimism and denial as coping strategies than those who accepted reality. However, to reiterate the risk of supporting optimism in your prognosis, if denial expressed as hope interferes with the patient realizing death as an eventuality, then the patient's behavior leaves them unprepared for the possibility of death. Avoiders conduct prognostic interviews with the intention of trying to limit or manipulate the patient's emotional reaction. These types of physicians typically experience the most personal discomfort around high intensity situations and have the most trouble communicating with patients. Because they feel ill-equipped to say the right thing, they avoid discussion by saying, "I don't know" when the patient asks for more information.

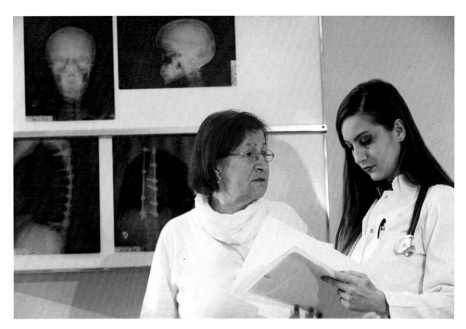

Avoiders also tend to shorten the length of the medical interview, leaving the patient with incomplete knowledge and a sense of confusion and isolation. Avoiding emotional encounters may lessen the physician's discomfort, but only increases patient dissatisfaction with the medical provider. Even if your intention is to reduce the patient's suffering and level of misdirected anger at you, the patient still will become angry at the way you avoided the situation.

## Determining How Much Patients Want to Know

One way to determine how much the patient wants to know is to have the patient fill out a question prompt list, so you have their information disclosure preferences before the first consultation. Many times, how-

ever, patients will broach the topic of prognosis before you do, sometimes in the form of a buried question or statement whereby they are
indirectly prompting you to speak about prognosis. Spotting the buried
question takes awareness of nonverbal cues, but if you become aware
of its presence, you can respond by exploring the buried question with
some of the responses outlined in Chapter 3. While using empathic
statements and open questions work to explore these cues, directly asking how much information the patient wants may not be the optimal
approach, as it can sometimes seem like a generic question. Some may
want a wide range of small details while others may want to focus on
the bigger picture.

When patients signal a desire for information, propose a number of different ways to answer the patient's questions rather than directly asking
how much information the patient wants. You might say, "I can answer
your question in several ways, so tell me which one is best for you," and
then run through a list of possible discussions until the patient signals a
preference. Once you begin providing information, remember to chunk
the information in digestible pieces so the patient can react to the information. If the patient indicates that they do not want to discuss prognostic information, try to explore the reasons why using the responses
outlined in Chapter 3. If further exploration indicates a fixable underlying reason, acknowledge the patient's concerns and ask permission to
revisit the topic at some point in the future. If the patient continues to
refuse all discussion of prognosis, make an assessment as to whether
disclosure of prognosis might improve the patient's ability to make decisions. If you cannot find a compelling reason to think it will improve
decision-making, follow the patient's wishes. If you believe information
disclosure may improve decision-making, ask the patient for permission
to disclose information with the family, as relatives may help the patient
avoid making poor decisions. If the patient refuses, start negotiating for

limited disclosure and explain why you think the patient would benefit from limited disclosure.

# Estimating Prognosis

Patients frequently ask physicians to estimate timelines for illness trajectories, whether they are chronic or temporary. Any estimate of prognosis should come with an explanation of the limitations in forecasting. This may require using the data collected by the physician, and translating it into plain language the patient can understand (i.e. formatting). When giving the patient a statistical, quantitative estimate of their illness trajectory timeline, researchers recommend using median (survival) rates and interquartile ranges (25th to 75th percentile) of a data set to convey prognosis. Researchers consider anything outside the interquartile range a prognosis extreme where only rare cases exist. The risk of giving a prognosis extreme, however likely, leaves open the possibility for inaccurate forecasting that the patient may come to resent or lead them to believe you have inaccurately forecasted the illness trajectory. Similarly, if you forgo the recommended range and give the patient an endpoint estimate such as, "You have six months," you risk credibility in the eyes of the patient if he or she lives longer than that endpoint. If you tell the patient they have roughly six months and the patient physically declines well before your prognostic endpoint, they will die feeling robbed of time. If you say, "I don't know" to avoid these risks, you may wind up heightening the patient's emotional uncertainty, leaving them vulnerable to fear and anxiety. Telling a patient with a serious, life-threatening illness that you do not know how long they may live also impedes determination of eligibility criteria for specific palliative care services. It limits the use of your expertise and prevents the patient and family from planning their agenda. Instead of using endpoints, give the interquartile range estimate, and use the 10th and 90th percentiles as a discussion for best- and worst-case scenarios. As such, doctors who accurately calculate forecasts make several considerations, which include:

- Whether the illness is typically associated with a poor or good prognosis (e.g. pancreatic cancer, biliary tract cancers, metastatic adenocarcinomas, untreated small cell lung cancers, etc.)

- What the specific functional declines are typically associated with the illness (e.g. progressive renal insufficiency, hyperkalemia, bone marrow failure, etc.)

- Illnesses that show momentum in their functional decline (rapid changes tend to continue rapidly, slow changes tend to continue slowly, and final stages tend to occur quickly)

Discussion of prognosis also may include an explanation of general momentum trends that the patient can watch for. For example, you might tell them that if functional decline increases momentum from month-to-month, it will likely continue for a number of months, but if functional decline increases momentum weekly, it is likely to continue for a number of weeks. Daily functional decline may indicate a prognosis limited to days.

According to Cornelius Woelk of the Regional Health Authority in Central Manitoba, studies show that performance status is an important predictor of survival, and that preexisting disease, prior treatment, psychological status, and social support may factor into the length of survival of patients with terminal illness. To this end, researchers designed the Karnofsky Performance Scale Index to classify patients according to their functional impairment, and to assess the prognosis in individual patients. The lower the Karnofsky score, the worse the survival for most serious illnesses. The table below illustrates the scale and criteria. Researchers have since modified the scale with the palliative performance scale, designed to measure physical status in palliative care. Using the palliative performance scale, a doctor would expect only about 10 percent of patients with a score of 50 percent or less to survive more than six months. For information on the palliative performance scale, see Appendix G.

*Table 1. Karnofsky Performance Scale*

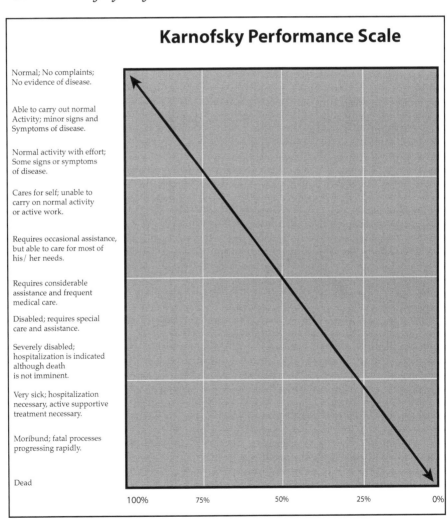

# Karnofsky Performance Scale

Normal; No complaints;
No evidence of disease.

Able to carry out normal
Activity; minor signs and
Symptoms of disease.

Normal activity with effort;
Some signs or symptoms
of disease.

Cares for self; unable to
carry on normal activity
or active work.

Requires occasional assistance,
but able to care for most of
his/ her needs.

Requires considerable
assistance and frequent
medical care.

Disabled; requires special
care and assistance.

Severely disabled;
hospitalization is indicated
although death
is not imminent.

Very sick; hospitalization
necessary, active supportive
treatment necessary.

Moribund; fatal processes
progressing rapidly.

Dead

| 100% | 75% | 50% | 25% | 0% |

# Outcomes of Discussing Prognosis

Whichever way you frame your prognosis, it is important to keep in mind the potential outcomes of your prognosis, as studies indicate that patients are more likely to volunteer for clinical trials or riskier treatments when prognosis for serious medical news is presented in a more positive light. A more positive type of disclosure may be one that focuses more on chances of surviving, while a more negative disclosure may be one that focuses more on chances of dying. Furthermore, the patient is more likely to seek longer-term benefits the more time you put into exploring the patient's emotions, concerns, and preferences in the prognostic interview. Treatment adherence is another outcome to consider in your approach to discussing prognosis. Therefore, if your treatment adherence factors into your clinical agenda, your discussion of prognosis about potential risks and benefits should include a conversation about statistical outcomes of adherence versus the statistical outcomes of non-adherence.

# Current and Historical Practices in Disclosing Bad News

Before the 1970s, physicians practicing medicine in the western world rarely told patients about their diagnosis and prognosis. However, as medical treatments improved and social attitudes on autonomy sparked legislative changes to informed consent, doctors increased their communication and expanded their disclosure methods. A combination of these factors shifted current practices in medicine toward patient-centered approaches whereby the right to self-determination now takes precedence over all other clinical considerations. Under the right to self-determination, doctors must place their patients at the center of the decision-making process by observing the practice of informed consent. The American Medical Association defines informed consent as a process of communication between a patient and physician that results in the patient's authorization or agreement to undergo a specific medical intervention. See Chapter 8 for further discussion on informed consent.

While most western cultures have adopted patient-centered approaches to medicine, non-western cultures still operate under family-centered approaches whereby doctors typically reveal diagnosis and prognosis to the family before the patient, and are required to withhold diagnosis and prognosis from the patient if the family requests it. According to the *Handbook of Communication in Oncology and Palliative Care*, "patients in Italy, China, Japan, Spain, Tanzania, Korea, and Mexico believe in a culturally determined value inherent in nondisclosure of diagnosis and terminal prognosis. This family-centered model of decision-making sees autonomy as isolating, cruel, and insensitive. Patients from an Egyptian background believe that dignity, identity, and security are conferred by belonging to a family; illness is managed by the family... in Taiwan, families believe that patients can be happier without knowing the truth." The family-centered approach may seem anomalous to western societies because informing the patient's family without consent of the patient would violate the patient's autonomy under the patient-centered approach. The reasons a patient may want to withhold information — as we will explore in Chapter 6 — may include an interfamilial conflict of interest, disagreement over treatment goals, or pre-existing relationship conflicts.

# How Structure and Content Influences Patient Recall

Since the predominant approach to managed care in western societies involves patient autonomy, how you structure the content of your consultations must directly influence a patient's comprehension and recall of information. With the goal of recall and comprehension in mind, your ability to organize the information must draw from three communication techniques: previewing the information, summarizing the information, and reviewing the next steps. Before you begin providing information, preview it by giving the patient an overview of the main points that you are about to cover. Consider the following scenario: You have just finished negotiating the amount of prognosis the patient wants you to disclose. Now you are about to give the prognosis, so you preview the information by saying, "Now that we've agreed to talk about survival rates for non-small cell lung cancer, I am going to talk about the median survival rate among people at stage IIA, and after that we can talk about the treatments you wanted to know about."

Studies show that patients retain information better when the emotional temperature is contained, so you might preface the prognosis by balancing reality with hope. For example, the prognosis for non-small cell lung cancer is typically better than the prognosis for small-cell lung cancer, so you might use your knowledge of this to offer the patient some hope and preserve their rate of retention. After providing information on stage IIA survival rates, you summarize by recapping the main details of the discussion, such as the symptoms of Stage IIA non-small cell lung cancer, the average life span of treated patients vs. untreated patients, the treatment options discussed, the treatment option your patient has chosen, and its regimen cycle. Follow your summary with checking behaviors as necessary (checking the patient for understanding, medical knowledge, and agenda preferences), and then review the next steps by telling the patient what he or she should do next. By going over the next steps, you make sure that you and the patient are on the same page. Combining content organization with checking skills helps the patient digest larger amounts of information and increases recall. By increasing recall, you avoid problems that result from poor memory retention, such as having the patient apply incorrect treatment dosages.

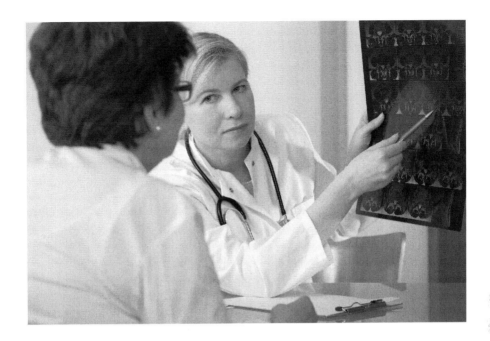

The process of creating a mentally organized structure that helps an individual acquire, code, store, recall, and decode information is called a cognitive map, a term coined by Edward Tolman in 1948. Most theoretical models and protocols previously discussed in this book are cognitive maps since they follow a structure designed to enhance patient autonomy as an outcome. The SPIKES protocol, devised by Robert Buckman, is another cognitive map that structures information with the goal of enhancing patient understanding and recall. Similar to the NURSE protocol, the SPIKES protocol exists as an acronym (**S**etup, **P**erception, **I**nvitation, **K**nowledge, **E**motion, and **S**ummarize). Chronologically, you would prepare for the conversation with the patient, assess the patient's perception of the illness, ask for an invitation to talk about the information, disclose the news in a straightforward manner, respond to the patient's emotion, and then summarize the plan. The last step in the SPIKES protocol ties together all the information discussed during the consultation and prepares the patient for the next steps. The SPIKES protocol recommends giving a brief written outline of the discussion to the patient and family to enhance recall and save time in the future by reducing confusion about what has already been discussed and agreed upon.

# Disclosing Clinical Errors

The occurrence of medical error is another form of negative medical news doctors must discuss frequently, and how you handle these errors can have an enormous impact on the entire medical institution. Due to the unpredictable nature of adverse outcomes, making a diagnosis or prognosis carries certain inherent risks, especially when an adverse outcome leads the patient to permanent injury or disability. Research shows that physicians disclose only one-third of all clinical errors to patients out of fear that full disclosure might lead to malpractice suits. If a doctor does disclose a clinical error, they may try to hide the mistake by confusing the patient with complex terminology. However, it is worth distinguishing clinical errors caused by mistakes in physician care from prognostic or diagnostic inaccuracies that result from external factors, such as a patient who withholds medical information, the body's individual response to treatment, or a disease that behaves uniquely to the individual. Due to increasing legislative trends and research indicating that a majority of adverse events are not the result of medical error, physicians should strive toward open disclosure.

## *Legal Implications and Trends in Disclosure*

Citing fear of litigation as a medical institution barrier to issuing disclosure and formal apologies, Australia, Canada, England, and states in the U.S. have responded by enacting "disclosure and apology laws." Disclosure laws mandate disclosure of serious unanticipated outcomes while apology laws provide institutions with a protective measure against plaintiffs using apologies as evidence of liability. While the limitations of study on litigation include factors unrelated to medical care (such as the patient's willingness to sue and attorneys willingness to negotiate settlements), studies show that open disclosure of medical error actually reduces the number of malpractice claims, time to resolution, and payouts. According to a 1999 study published by Steve Kraman and Ginny Hamm in the *Annals of Internal Medicine*, "When a malpractice claim is made against an institution in the private sector, risk managers coordinate the defense against patients, their dependents, and their attorneys. The medical institution and the patient often become adversaries, and patients and attorneys frequently seek punitive as well as loss-based damages...anger at a perceived betrayal of trust is part of the patients' motivation." Likewise, Gerald Hickson's 1992 study in the *Journal of the American Medical Association* revealed that, "Of 127 families who sued their health care providers after perinatal injuries, 43 percent were motivated by the suspicion of a cover-up or by the desire for revenge."

When medical institutions honestly admit medical errors and offer timely, comprehensive help in filing claims, plaintiffs and their attorneys statistically become more willing to negotiate smaller settlements as opposed to filing for larger punitive judgments. The National Quality Forum provides safe practice disclosure guidelines and reveals a growing trend toward open disclosure as it correlates to reduced malpractice suits. In 2005, it reported that at least 70 percent of all health care organizations had established disclosure policies. To model your disclosure policies to a national standard, go to **www.qualityforum.org/Home. aspx**. The components of institutional disclosure under Safe Practice include protocols for conducting a formal apology, disclosure coaching and training for medical staff, and emotional support for patients and health care practitioners involved in adverse, unexpected outcomes. The *Handbook of Communication in Oncology and Palliative Care* recommends four steps in communicating error disclosure to patients.

## Step 1

Seek the help of institutional resources such as patient safety analysts and quality officers. After an error is uncovered, the emotional distress of the medical staff may affect its ability to recall how the error occurred as well as its ability to deliver negative medical news to the patient in a calm and positive fashion.

## Step 2

Plan the initial disclosure of error with the medical staff. Arrange a meeting with the medical staff involved in the error to discuss how the error occurred, the questions you expect to answer, and how to rectify the error. At the end of the meeting, assign team members their roles for the entire process.

## Step 3

Conduct the error disclosure with the patient. You should hold this conversation within 24 hours of your discovery of the error. Using the CONES protocol, safe practice guidelines, or related theoretical model of breaking bad news, provide information about the adverse outcome and its health implications for the patient, as well as what steps the staff has taken to rectify the problem.

## Step 4

Use an institutional risk manager to conduct a follow-up conversation with the patient. This conversation should provide an opportunity to discuss any new discoveries regarding the nature of error and the steps taken to safeguard the patient's health in the future. In some cases, the nature of the error may have nothing to do with clinical error on the part of the medical staff, but rather, external factors attributing to the error. In this instance, the follow-up conversation serves as a means of letting the patient know that the institution has conducted its due diligence in the interest of patient safety and uncovered no sign of negligence on the part of the medical staff. If the risk manager reveals an error on the part of the medical staff, a formal apology is necessary.

## Other Types of Prognostic Errors and Influences

University of Chicago professor Nicholas A. Christakis conducted a study of terminal patients, which found a number of additional factors that influenced prognostic errors. While the study indicated no important difference in prognostic errors relating to age, sex, race, religion, or marital status, empirical evidence showed prognostic errors were influenced by the length of the doctor-patient relationship, the time since last examination, the physician's sub-specialty training, general over-optimism over specific diseases, and general over-pessimism of specific diseases. Unexpected deterioration is also a type of prognostic error physicians must account for. To address this communication challenge, researchers recommend using the CONES protocol outlined on the next page. Prognostic errors also may result from lack of access to patient information, inadequate documentation, and inconsistent practices among health professionals providing care to a patient. However, one of the most common influences of prognostic error involves medication related to cytotoxic drugs. No matter how clearly you outline a treatment regimen, an adverse outcome is likely to occur if the patient inaccurately doses on the prescribed medication, thereby rendering your prognosis inaccurate, if only by appearance. Technically, this qualifies as an external factor related to prognostic error, but the error requires an explanation nonetheless. To avoid inaccurate treatment dosage, written information should cover the following aspects of medication:

- Name of medication and purpose
- Storage requirements
- Dose and duration of therapy
- Potential side effects and precautions
- What to do in the event of dosage error
- Possible toxic reactions and methods for prevention
- Potential effects of interaction with foods, other drugs, and other diseases

# Conducting System Failure Analysis

In 1999, the Institute of Medicine released a report that significantly increased awareness of medical errors and highlighted the need for reliable data on the number of medical errors occurring in health care facilities. Today, many medical institutions rely on web-based surveillance systems to track medical errors. A systems failure analysis is an investigation to determine the underlying reasons for errors, and to recommend appropriate corrective actions. To conduct system failure analysis of medical errors, health care practitioners have adopted the failure mode and effect analysis (FMEA) system, illustrated in Figure 8, which outlines a five-step protocol as a preventative measure to reduce error.

**Step 1**

Define and identify topics that potentially caused the medical errors and compartmentalize them into high-risk, high-severity, high-probability categories.

## Step 2

Assemble a team consisting of multidisciplinary personnel from different backgrounds with expertise in matters related to the topics you have identified as potentially causes of the medical error. Call upon these subject matter experts to investigate the potential causes surrounding the medical error and allow them to provide insight into their findings.

## Step 3

Develop and consult a visual process map that the team can follow as a protocol for conducting a system failure analysis. This protocol should include all the process tasks required to execute Steps 1-5, including investigative methods and instructions for reporting.

## Step 4

Conduct hazard analysis as a means of refining and improving process tasks.

## Step 5

Develop a corrective action that addresses the error to ensure the patient's future safety.

*Figure 8. Failure Mode and Effect Analysis System*

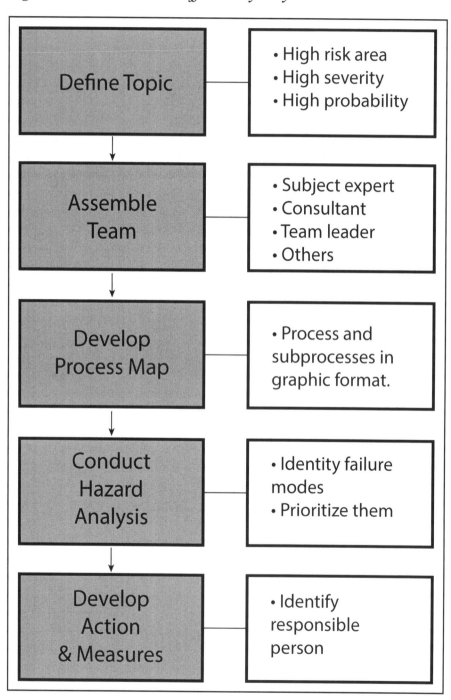

# The CONES Approach

Disclosing medical error is a unique form of breaking negative medical news because you are obligated to let the patient know that an error has occurred as opposed to giving the patient the option of hearing the news. For this reason, researchers designed the SPIKES protocol for optional discussions and the CONES protocol for disclosing error. Like its predecessor, the CONES protocol stands as an acronym (Context, Opening remark, Narrative, Emotions, Strategy and summary). Context refers to getting the physical context of the situation right. Physical factors include the handshake, sitting at the same eye level of the patient, and establishing a calm demeanor. Other positive physical contexts to adopt include creating a neutral posture, maintaining a distance of about three to five feet from the patient, smiling, and leaning forward. The opening remark establishes who you are and sets the agenda. If someone has already informed the patient of the error, it is helpful to issue your apology as the opening remark. If not, proceed with introductions. Once you establish context and make your opening remark, your narrative should start at the beginning of the condition, highlight how the condition looked to the medical staff at the time, and give a chronological account of the events surrounding the error. Afterwards, explain how you discovered the error, the steps taken to investigate the error, the conclusions made by your staff, and corrective measures taken to rectify or prevent the error in the future. Along the way, stop at various intervals to respond to any reactions emoting from the patient and offer the opportunity for questions. The narrative should be an honest account of the situation. While it is not recommended to say "I don't know" when giving a prognosis, it is acceptable to admit that you do not know an answer to the discussion of medical error, but that you promise to try and find the answer to the patient's question. When it comes to dealing with emotions, acknowledge the emotions and their cause, using an empathic statement or any of the responding techniques covered earlier. After you have allowed the patient to express their emotional reactions to the news, arrange to contact the patient and provide a phone number, as this will increase goodwill. For further information on formal apologies, go to **www.sorryworks.net**.

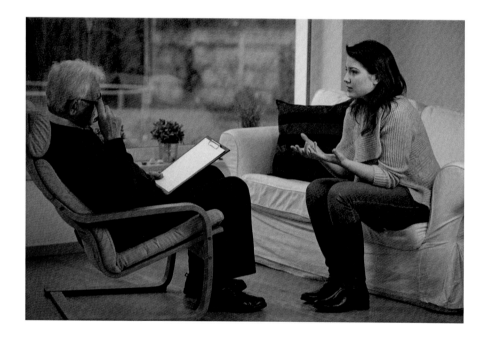

# Chapter 5

# How to Support Patient Decision-making

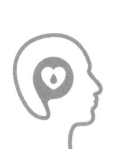

R esearch into the practical application of supporting patient decision-making has become a topic of widespread discussion over the last 20 years. The ancient Greeks believed that the physician's primary task was to win the confidence of the patient. They considered informing the patient a sign of uncertainty and lack of expertise. During medieval times, doctors were encouraged to manipulate medical discussions as a way of offering comfort and hope. By the 1880s, arguments over informed consent began to challenge the medical profession over whether patients should actively participate in decisions regarding their medical treatment.

Today, research studies show that about 92 percent of patients want information about their illness and treatment options. Before the 1980s, the paternalistic model of decision-making still dominated. As the paternalistic model waned, a more informed and consumer-oriented model of decision-making became the preferred clinical approach to consultation. For example, in 1961, 90 percent of doctors surveyed revealed that they preferred not to disclose a cancer diagnosis. In 1979, 97 percent of doctors surveyed revealed that they preferred telling their patients that they had cancer. So, what changed between 1961 and 1979? The answer lies in the rise of treatment options, improved curability, and Western society's culture shift toward self-determination as a right.

While most doctors today prefer full (or at least partial) disclosure, patients do not unanimously agree. In a 2010 *American Journal of Managed Care* study published by Lesley Degner, "roles in treatment decision-making that patients preferred were 26 percent active, 49 percent collaborative, and 25 percent passive… only 6 percent experienced extreme discordance [with their physician] between their preferred versus actual roles." According to Degner, many investigations have shown that higher education and occupational skill level is associated with preference for a more active role. Despite any debate that may still exist over which model better serves the patient, the important issue is determining how to figure out what the patient needs.

# Paternalistic Model

Three types of decision-making models exist in clinical application: the paternalistic model, the informed model, and the shared model. Given the nature of today's accepted practice of determining how much information the patient wants, some physicians may blur the lines between models by using a combination of theoretical approaches. To this end, Lesley Degner introduced a conceptual model that places decision-making approaches along a spectrum that ranges from paternalistic to patient-centered. In their purest form, three conceptual models exist. Thus, a visual representation of the spectrum would appear as overlapping models. The paternal and informed models represent opposite extremes, with the shared decision-making model representing the median model, as shown in Figure 9.

*Figure 9. Spectrum of Decision-Making Models*

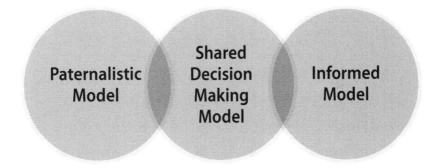

The paternalistic model is the clinical approach used by most physicians before 1980. Under the paternalistic model, the physician imparts information to the patient as the physician sees fit and makes treatment recommendations without offering options. The patient passively receives the information and agrees to treatment recommendations. The paternalistic model omits discussions about the patient's agenda beyond treatment and cure, as well as their preferences with respect to treatment outcomes, and techniques used by the physician to elicit a two-way dialogue. Four assumptions guide the decision-making process in the paternalistic approach: the doctor is well trained and educated, the doctor is in the best position to choose the most effective treatment, other doctors would make the same recommendations, and all the doctor's decisions are guided by concern for the patient's health.

# The Informed Model

In contrast to the paternalistic model, the informed model sits on the other end of Degner's shared decision-making spectrum. Under the informed model, the patient is the sole decision maker and the physician plays the role of information provider. As the information provider, the physician discloses information according to patient preferences and then communicates all treatment options, including their risks and benefits so that the patient can make an informed choice. If your patient prefers to make decisions via the informed model, your discussions must include any information relevant to enhancing the patient's decision-making process. The physician acts as an agent, executing the management plan on behalf of the patient's wishes and decisions. The patient predominantly directs a one-way dialogue during clinical interviews while the physician listens and waits for the patient to request more information. Because patients control the flow of the information exchange, most of the discussion will be medical in nature rather than personal. Under this model, the patient is likely to volunteer personal information as a means of aiding their decision. You should avoid eliciting personal information unless the patient signals a desire to discuss it.

# The Shared Decision-Making Model

Under the shared decision-making model, both patients and doctors mutually collaborate to access relevant information to enable patient-centered selection of health care resources. This doctor-patient relationship interaction occurs throughout each stage of the decision-making process whereby the physician communicates evidence-based information about treatment options, as well as their risks and benefits. While the informed model discourages the physician from eliciting a conversation about personal information, the shared decision-making model encourages information seeking of this kind. Here, you may inquire about the patient's values, lifestyle, and preferences in order to recommend and negotiate treatment options based on the patient's answers and your clinical values. Because the shared decision-making model overlaps into some of the features of its two counterparts, it therefore serves as the most common and recommended approach to supporting patient decision-making in today's medical environment. The shared decision-making process allows both parties to express their opinion about treatment preferences. Keep in mind, however, that most patients expect patient-centered service, so if the patient rejects your treatment preferences after lengthy negotiations, you ultimately will have to accept and execute the patient's agenda. If the patient's agenda violates ethical practice, you must inform the patient of your ethical duty to reject it (for more on ethical issues, see Chapter 8).

Of the three decision-making models, the shared decision-making model offers the most opportunity to implement some of the techniques discussed in this book. Proponents of shared decision-making argue that physicians are best suited to collect relevant data on the patient's condition, and patients are best suited to make the decisions that weigh with values and trade-offs according to preference and need. Collaborative decision-making thus leads to improvements in the treatment relationship and health outcomes. According to a 2006 study published in the *Community Mental Health Journal* by Jared Adams and Robert Drake, "Some advocates for shared decision-making believe that increased client choice will lead not only to improved client outcomes but also to reduced costs, because ineffective treatments will be used less often." However, not all patients prefer or enjoy making the decisions. In this instance, the shared model may actually work at cross-purposes with the clinical agenda and patient satisfaction. For some patients, too many choices can debilitate the patient and increase their sense of lost opportunity if they wind up regretting their treatment choices.

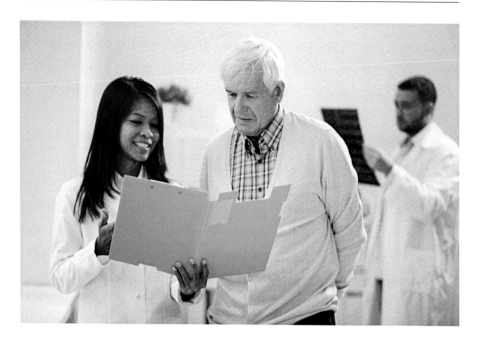

Because physicians commonly fail to explore patient preferences in decision-making, evidence on shared decision-making and clinical outcomes remains mixed. Potential barriers may prevent physicians from using the shared decision-making model altogether. For example, if the doctor has insufficient data after the first consultation, they may feel ill-equipped to make sound recommendations and choices regarding the management plan. In other cases, the patient's health may pose certain barriers. For instance, if the patient has other health problems, the treatments you recommend may create additional health complications. Sometimes other specialists create decision-making barriers when they give the patient conflicting information about the treatments you recommended.

## Exploring Patient Preferences in Decision-Making

Studies show that physicians make roughly 70 to 80 percent of all primary care diagnoses based on patients' reported medical history. As the physician, you must determine the patient's preferences in decision-making participation through information provision. The physician should engage in specific exploratory behaviors, which include:

- Asking more questions to understand the client's problems, expectations, and perspectives
- Exploring the patient's reported medical history with regard to symptoms, occurrence, and past treatments
- Encouraging the client to ask more questions
- Giving clear information
- Showing support and empathy
- Explaining the patient's decision-making options (paternal, informed, shared)
- Recommending the shared decision-making model if the patient expresses interest in participating in the decision-making process

If the patient signals an unwillingness to make any decisions, try to explore the reasons for their preference, as further inquiry may reveal fixable, emotional barriers preventing the patient from choosing a more beneficial preference. According to studies by Adams and Drake, "Adherence [to participation] was sometimes related to communication variables. Clients who felt they had expressed themselves fully and received all the information they wanted had better functional outcomes. Client satisfaction was most closely linked to the practitioner's ability to display concern, warmth, and interest." When previewing the range of decision-making options available, categorize or code decisions into potential outcomes, impact on lifestyle, employment, relationships, and family life. This gives the patient an understanding as to the gravity of each decision so that the patient can see the relationship between choice and consequence, and how much control they want over that relationship. If possible, draw diagrams to illustrate a surgical technique or outcome from a treatment approach.

# Classification of Intervention Intensity

Patients need more than the ability to ask questions; they need to know how to express what is important to them. To determine decision-making preference, the physician must choose an intervention intensity as an approach to discussion preferences. Intervention intensities exist in three varying degrees: low, moderate, and high. In a low-intensity intervention, the doctor offers little verbal guidance, and instead provides written visual aids that explain potential outcomes to treatment and encourages the patient to ask questions. Moderate-intensity interventions involve multimedia presentations that explain decision-making outcomes in greater detail. The presentation encourages the patient to formulate questions based on the material, which assists the patient in articulating preferences to the physician. High-intensity interventions involve educating the patient about models of communication skills, such as videos of patients expressing preferences, role-playing exercises, and explicit verbal guidance from a health educator or the physician. Research of high-, low-, and moderate-intensity interventions show that high-intensity interventions are more effective in aiding patient preferences in decision-making.

# Exploring the Patient's Personal History

Exploring the patient's medical history is one of the key components of information provision. In order to determine whether the patient is mentally and physically able to participate in decision-making, you must form a picture of their previous medical history. The medical history should involve not just the physical symptoms of dysfunction, but also the individual's perspective on the symptoms. The goal of exploring the patient's personal history is to increase your understanding of the patient's background and its impact on the problem for which the patient has sought help. To this end, researchers recommend using a combination of open-ended and closed questions. The goal of medical history recording, therefore, involves seeking answers to five questions.

- Which organs are causing the symptoms?
- What is the likely cause?
- What are the risk factors?
- Are there any complications?
- What are the patient's ideas, concerns, and expectations?

Gaining insight into these questions requires exploration into family history, personal history, social history, past medical history, including possible drug and allergy history. Exploring family history may reveal evidence of inherited or genetic disorders, especially if the symptoms match. To begin the family and social history inquiry, ask if the patient has a regular sexual partner and if their partner reported any recent change in their health status. Next, ask if there are any children and get the age and state of health for each child, followed by an inquiry about near relatives who died and from what cause. Some physicians find it helpful to construct a family tree when taking notes on family history. A person's social history (i.e. their social relationships, sexual orientation, and emotional attachments) may have a bearing on the current condition. To gain insight into the patient's current condition, you must explore the possibility of major health inequalities resulting from social class and income. A detailed social history may include information provision about schooling, employment, social support networks, and leisure activities. Social history is particularly important for elderly patients, as their health status often depends on domestic and social support networks. Gathering these types of social data points provides a context for assessing the impact of diseases and disorders on intellectual and/or social function. Likewise, exploring employment history may provide insight into possible working conditions linked to the current condition, such as environmental exposure to hazardous materials. If the patient has traveled anywhere, note the locations and research possible diseases endemic to that location, which match the symptoms of the current condition. The patient's medical history should include health status before and after the onset of the problem.

Studies show that patients recall their medical history with varying degrees of detail and accuracy. Asking the patient about previous admittance to hospital for a procedure may jog their memory. Some patients have trouble recalling the names of their medications. To jog memory and compile accurate details, ask for the labeled bottles or a written list of medicines prescribed by the previous doctor. If the medical history is long and complicated, ask for old records and reports. If you suspect age and background as potential factors influencing the condition, use the communication techniques outlined in Chapter 2 to ask if the patient has experimented with recreational drugs. After completing the family and social medical history, conduct a biological systems review. A systems review can help you identify symptoms or concerns that patients may have failed to mention in their family or social history. It also can help you determine if a symptom is not an actual symptom of illness. A systems review of the body may include notes on:

- General symptoms
- Cardiovascular system
- Gastrointestinal system

- Genitourinary system
- Nervous system
- Musculoskeletal system
- A medical history summary

General health questions may include an exploration of sleeping patterns, weight loss, fevers, rashes, etc. If your previous line of questioning answered a question surrounding a particular organ, there is no need to cover a system review for that organ; simply indicate "see above" in your notes. For a medical case history sample, including a standard family tree, see Appendix H.

# Addressing Treatment Options

After you have completed a medical history profile and confirmed your diagnosis, ensuing discussions should focus on developing a management plan. If the patient has agreed to participate in the decision-making process, you must facilitate a discussion on which treatment option to choose. A skilled communicator structures key information into all aspects of this medical decision. After you have established a framework for the consultation and negotiated an agenda, introduce the concept of decision-making, recommend an approach based on the negotiated agenda, and ask the patient to choose. Since shared decision-making is the most recommended approach to managed care, and patient comprehension is vital to shared decision-making, you must use communication skills and process tasks to help the patient understand:

- The nature of the disease
- The benefits and risks of each treatment choice
- The implications of each treatment's potential outcome to the patient's life and negotiated agenda

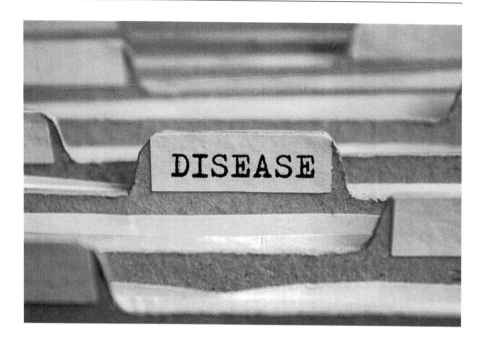

In order to meet these objectives, use process tasks, such as talking in non-technical language, drawing diagrams whenever possible, and categorizing the information into chunks so that the patient can delineate between treatments and avoid mixing up their benefits and risks. The communication skills required to complete these process tasks include having the ability to clearly preview and summarize information, checking for understanding after each explanation, and eliciting questions. To preview the information, you might start by saying, "First I'd like to preview and summarize the treatments available to you, and then we can talk about each of them." Eliciting questions about the treatment options should then lead to discussions about matching the patient's values and lifestyle factors in accordance with the benefits and risks presented with each treatment option. Process tasks used to match the patient's values and lifestyle factors include getting the patient to talk about the impact of potential treatment outcomes on self-image, employment, lifestyle, and personal relationships. The physician can accomplish this through the techniques outlined in this book, such as using open questions, empathic statements, validation of emotional response, and so forth. For example, you might ask, "What have you already learned about your treatment options?" / "Do any of your family members receive treatment for this illness?" / "Do you have any concerns or issues that might influence your decision?"

During this time, do not interrupt the patient to give them your recommendation. Let them finish, acknowledge their concerns, and then proceed with a statement that presents your treatment recommendation. For example, you might say, "If you were my relative, I would recommend that you go with treatment option x because..." This type of statement is empathic because it shows the patient that you are putting yourself in their position and showing what type of decision you would make if it were personal to you. In giving your recommendation, provide a clear and logical reason for why you believe it is the best available option. Expressing confidence in the treatment plan also will help ease the patient's concerns about the potential outcomes. Once you have finished, summarize what you have said, ask open questions, and offer the patient a chance to take a few days to think about the options before deciding. For example, you might say, "Now that you understand the treatment options, I just want to make sure you understand what I've recommended for you..." / "If you're not up to making a decision today, you can take a few days to think it over..." If the patient decides upon a treatment option, arrange for consent forms, as well as additional consultations or referrals, and create a plan detailing the next steps in the process of health management. For example, you might say, "Okay, let me tell you about the next steps. First, you need to sign a consent form for the treatment option. You have to make an appointment for this at the front desk. Once you sign the forms, we will get you started on the management plan..." If the patient decides to delay the decision and has no other questions, close the consultation, remind them of your availability, and tell them you look forward to speaking again.

# Road Map for Involving Patients in Decision-Making

When it comes to involving patients in the decision-making process, physicians must avoid overwhelming them with information about treatment options when they may already feel overwhelmed by the emotional overtones of life-and-death scenarios. For this reason, the road map for involving patients in decision-making involves:

- Preparing for the consultation
- Framing the decision
- Asking for the patient's preferences
- Outlining options under the shared decision-making approach
- Outlining options under the paternalistic approach
- Checking for patient comprehension
- Establishing the patients preference for decision-making

The only way to express confidence about treatment options is to know everything about the treatment options. Resist the impulse to think aloud, as it may create the impression that you are not certain about something. If you say that you do not know something about the treatment, you may appear disengaged, uncommitted to your profession, or incompetent. Therefore, make sure that you have a firm command of information when it comes to treatment options and how it relates to the patient's problem. When you frame the decision, you must clearly describe the decision the patient must make. To frame the decision, you present the problem and the possibility of choices. For example, you might say something like, "Since your heart valve is narrowed, the issue we need to decide is whether or not you should have aortic stenosis surgery." A discussion can start by summarizing key findings in the medical history you recorded. In this discussion, you would determine decision-making preferences and then outline the options according to the decision-making model chosen by the patient (paternal, informed, shared). If the patient prefers the shared or informed approach, explain that there is a lot of information to cover and encourage the patient to speak up if they become confused, review the pros and cons of each treatment, and offer a recommendation. If the patient prefers the paternal approach, make a recommendation and offer your rationale for why you believe it is the best option. Along the way, you check for comprehension by asking the patient to summarize what you have said. Finally, determine how the patient wants to proceed, describe the next steps of the management plan, and close the consultation.

# Using Decision-Making Aids

Facilitating the decision-making process can be difficult with patients who are not certain about their preferences. When it comes to patients who demonstrate this type of irresolution, decision-making aids can reduce conflict and increase patient satisfaction. Generally, patients feel more comfortable if they are fully informed, but may respond to different types of materials, so if you provide your patient with decision-making aids, be sure to have a variety of formats available. Decision-making aid formats include:

- Handwritten summary
- Literature (brochures, workbooks and handouts)
- Photos (visual aids)
- Interactive computer programs and decision-board simulators
- Audio tapes
- Coach-based management and value clarification exercises

Some formats require home use; others involve participation between the physician and patient during the consultation. No matter which format you choose to provide, it should address both physical and psychosocial concerns, the different types of clinical decision-making, the trade-offs between risks and benefits associated with treatments, and the role of all parties involved. Written materials, however, may not answer all of the patient's questions, so you might consider asking a current or former patient who has gone through a similar circumstance if they would be willing to speak with the patient. Should they agree to consult, this person may share personal experiences that help the deciding patient choose their preference. The simplest decision aid is the brief summary (roughly 1 page long) handwritten by the physician while talking to the patient. The handwritten summary should consist of a basic outline of the conversation, listing the diagnosis, stage of illness (if applicable), patient values, treatment options, anticipated outcomes, and possible side effects to each organ system.

The audio recording is the second simplest aid. This aid not only assists patient comprehension, but also helps family members understand the range of choices if they were not present during the consultation. However, if the emotional temperature of the patient appears heightened, consider the handwritten option, as an audio recording may recreate distress for the patient when replayed. Decision aids also carry a number of general assumptions about decision-making that may distort or appear inconsistent with the way the individual patient usually makes decisions. The range of assumptions may include established cultural beliefs, ethical precepts, medical paradigms, and concepts of risk. The physician, therefore, should make the patient aware of such assumptions before recommending any aids. If you consider using decision aids in your practice and are unsure of what constitutes an effective decision aid, you can measure the quality of decision aids by using the internationally approved set of criteria established by the International Patient Decision Aid Standards Collaboration (IPDAS). This group consists of more than 100 researchers, medical practitioners, and patients from 14 countries. To compare the quality of decision aids, IPDAS examines the differences in clinical content, and the development process, as well as the aid's reported effect on patient decisions, burden, conflict, regret, anxiety, depression, health status, and quality of life.

Keep in mind that while decision aids tend to increase knowledge and acquisition of treatment options, they statistically have not shown a significant impact on lowering anxiety or conflict, according to a study published by Mary Ann O'Brien in the *Journal of Clinical Oncology*. To measure the quality of your decision aids beyond the reports provided by IPDAS, assess whether the choice the patient made (using the decision aid) was consistent with the values they expressed during the clinical interview.

# Using Clinical Experience to Support Decision-Making

Whether your patients choose to participate in decision-making or leave all the decisions in your hands, patients do not have the benefit of clinical knowledge when they make choices. For example, if a patient wants to order a certain test that you believe is a waste of money, consider offering your opinion, using examples from your clinical experience to explain why you believe this. Offering an opinion based on your clinical experience is different from making a medical recommendation on treatment options. In the case of the former, you are offering an option for dealing with chronic illness beyond the options presented. The roadmap for using your clinical experience to support decision-making requires four steps. First, ask the patient about their perspective on the symptom or concern. Even if their perspective is clinically inaccurate, addressing the perspective is the first step toward using clinical experience to guide the patient. Second, use the empathic or NURSE statement to comment on the emotional content surrounding the issue. Let the patient reflect on the statement and then offer your opinion as a hypothesis. For example, you might say, "It sounds like you're a little afraid that if we don't run all the tests then there's something we might miss here. I see a lot of patients in your position who get tests they do not need because of this understandable fear, but in my experience, this test is not necessary and will not tell us anything." After you offer your hypothesis, ask the patient if he or she would like to hear about other patients you treated with the same problem. The purpose of this is to offer alternate ways of approaching managed care beyond the options they might feel limited to. Do not impose your clinical experience; simply offer it. If the patient accepts your opinion, ask the patient if your opinion has given them a new perspective.

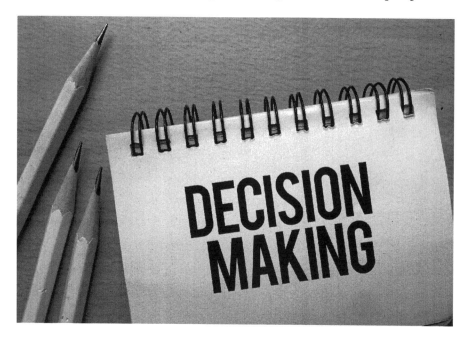

Checking for comprehension constitutes a portion of the information disclosure stage, as observed in theoretical models of communication such as the SEGUE framework and Calgary-Cambridge guide. Their level of comprehension also may indicate whether you have effectively translated technical jargon into plain, easy-to-understand language. For some physicians, this is the most difficult part of information sharing because technical jargon allows for the rapid exchange of information in time-crunch professions. Thus, having to translate technical jargon may be time consuming, especially for physicians who feel the pressure of limiting the duration of their interviews. Effective translation of technical terms also increases the patient's emotional satisfaction with the interview, and leads to greater symptom relief, functional and psychological status, and pain control.

In order to tackle the challenge of determining how much information you will have to translate, compile a list of technical terms you most commonly use in your clinical encounters and translate them into plain language that people without medical degrees would understand. Translating terms beforehand will save you from wasting time trying to find the right explanation. Since no two patients are alike in their level of technical understanding, be prepared to encounter patients who prefer technical jargon as well as patients who prefer plain translations. For example, patients well into an illness trajectory are more likely to understand technical jargon than those receiving bad news for the first time. Patients in the former category are more apt to have had many previous conversations with other physicians at that point. Other factors, such as ethnicity or socioeconomic status, may influence the physician's approach to medical jargon. Whichever the case, you must accommodate the patient's wishes, so before you see the patient, make a note of the technical terms relevant to your discussion and mentally rehearse your translations. Once you elicit the patient's story about the illness, listen to their description. The patient's vocabulary may provide a rough estimate as to their technical understanding of the problem. Do they use technical jargon or plain language? Once you have determined their level of technical understanding, adjust your translations accordingly. If you are not sure about the patient's level of proficiency after listening to them speak, conduct a test. Use a technical word, wait for a nonverbal cue that indicates understanding or confusion, and then translate it into plain language. Some patients may signal an understanding of the technical jargon and stop you from explaining, others may signal relief from their confusion. To get an idea of how translation works, Robert Buckman provides examples of technical terms translated into useful phrases in his book, *Difficult Conversations in Medicine*, listed in the table below. For a more comprehensive table of Buckman's translated terms, see Appendix I.

*Table 2. Translating Technical Ideas into Plain Language*

| The Technical Idea | Examples of Useful Phrases |
|---|---|
| Clinical Trial | Comparison of a new treatment with the standard one that everyone uses at the moment |
| Randomization | The electronic equivalent of flipping a coin so there is no bias as to who gets which treatment |
| Axillary Node Sampling | Taking some lymph nodes from the armpit to see if there has been any spread |
| Sentinel Node Biopsy | Taking just a few nodes nearest the breast |
| Neoadjuvant Therapy | Treatment given before surgery to try and shrink the tumor |

# Recommending Clinical Trials

After you have discussed all of the standard treatment options, you may consider offering your patient the option of enrolling in clinical trials. If you decide to offer this option as a possible decision, you should define the nature of a clinical trial by explaining the three types of phases. If you recommend a Phase I trial, explain that these are initial studies with limited enrollment with the purpose of evaluating dosage safety and the frequency and methods by which the potentially new drug should be administered. If you recommend a Phase II trial, explain that these are trials designed to evaluate drug and dosage safety, which zero in on very specific types of illnesses. If you recommend a Phase III trial, explain that this type of trial tests new drug combinations by comparing them against current standards of treatment. Naturally, since Phase I trials are the most experimental and unknown, patients may find them to be the most promising, so you should make your patient aware of the clinical trial status if you recommend one (see Chapter 8 for ethical concerns regarding enrollment in clinical trials). Recommendations for clinical trials should only begin after you have completed discussions of standard treatments. Using the SEGUE method, you can help your patients decide about clinical trials in five steps.

## Step 1

Present the clinical trial as an alternative treatment option. Describe the purpose and rationale of the clinical trial. Explain the risks and benefits by comparing the experimental treatment against the standard treatment.

**Step 2**

Provide the patient with an opportunity to talk about their understanding and attitude toward the clinical trial.

**Step 3**

Declare and emphasize your views on the trial as being an acceptable option, whether used alone or in combination with the standard treatment. Assure the patient that his or her choice will not affect the doctor-patient relationship or other staff assigned to their care.

**Step 4**

Offer the patient the opportunity to declare their decision regarding the clinical trial or take a few days to consider the option.

**Step 5**

If the patient declines the clinical trial, turn the discussion back to the standard treatment options. If the patient decides to defer the option for a later consultation, make a future appointment. If they agree to the clinical trial, initiate steps toward enrollment and describe the next steps for the patient.

# Communicating Survivorship

After you assist chronically ill patients with treatment decisions, they will need to make decisions about survivorship care. Creating a survivorship plan requires examination of long-term management after discharge from treatment. Researchers define survivorship at three points along the illness trajectory: at the time of diagnosis, during periods of remission, and long-term survival living with consequences of the disease. Survivorship issues may vary between different types of diseases, so you must examine the individual issues that you expect your patients will face, such as late- and long-term effects of treatment. Since late effects may include unrecognizable toxicities that manifest after the end of therapy and long-term effects include complications that occur during and after therapy, you must identify the key issues of survivorship, which include:

- Physical well-being
- Social well-being
- Psychosocial well-being
- Spiritual well-being

To support the patient's physical well-being, you must negotiate decisions that cover physical activities, strength, fatigue, and pain. To support social well-being, you must negotiate decisions that cover family issues, sexual function with a partner, confidence, employment, and finances. To support psychosocial well-being, you must negotiate decisions that cover anxiety, distress, depression, employment, and fear of recurrence. During the decision-making process, a survivorship plan should categorize all types of therapies and their possible late effects to every organ. Upon discharge of treatment, provide the patient with a record of all care received, as well as important disease characteristics, and include lifestyle guidelines for survivors. Discussion of late effects is perhaps the most important part of communicating survivorship because patients unaware of absent but potential manifestations are less prone to follow the recommendations of survivorship care. In order to execute the challenges posed in survivorship, researchers recommend helping the patient decide between three models of survival care delivery: Shared care, nurse-led care, and survivorship clinics.

Shared care places the responsibility of survivorship care on the primary care physician. Their role may include helping the patient through the physical and emotional aspects of survivorship, managing the aspects of chronic disease, handling specialist referrals, and consulting with specialists in cases of uncertainty. Nurse-led care places the responsibility of survivorship care on a team of nurses who coordinate all aspects of health management and handle specialist referrals. Survivorship clinics are specialized institutions that facilitate a coordinated approach to medical and psychosocial problems encountered by survivors. Roughly 35 of these clinics currently exist in the United States and are typically run by nurses trained in oncology, pediatric oncologists, and additional personnel specialists.

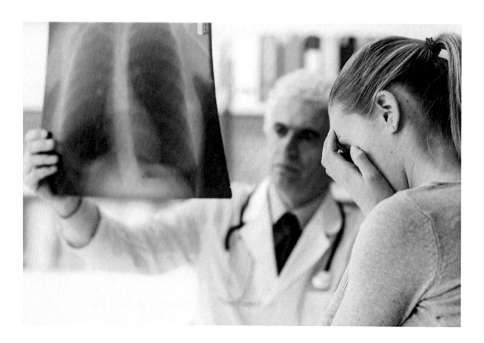

# Recognizing Patient Depression and Over-Dependency

For better or worse, the patient's decisions at various points in survivorship, both during and after treatment, will have consequences, and their reaction to those consequences may take the form of depression. Medical institutions have defined depression as a chronic state of lowered mood. To help a depressed patient, you will have to recognize the symptoms and the severity of the condition in order to provide support. Depressive symptoms listed in the *Diagnostic and Statistical Manual of Mental Disorders*, fourth edition (DSM-IV) include irritability, diminished interest in life activities, insomnia, psychomotor agitation, fatigue, feelings of worthlessness, lack of concentration, and recurring thoughts of suicide or death. If you identify depression as the cause of these symptoms, be prepared to treat depression by obtaining a psychiatric referral. During the survivorship stage, the patient may look to you continually for help with their problems. While you should be supportive, you also should look for signs of over-dependency. Over-dependency can be dangerous to the patient's welfare, to their coping strategies, and to your relationship because this behavior decreases the patient's abilities of self-determination. If the patent becomes over-dependent and their condition worsens, they may blame you for the outcome. Because depression manifests as loss of interest in decision-making, over-dependency may result. To address the problem of depression and over-dependency, researchers recommend three steps.

## Step 1

**Make the diagnosis.** Depression is a disorder with easily recognizable physical symptoms. Run through the list of symptoms provided above and determine if any are physically present.

## Step 2

**Make the patient aware of the depressive symptoms.** Align the patient's knowledge by first asking what he or she thinks the problem might be. Afterward, educate the patient about the facts of depression, and possibly draw on your clinical experience about what you have seen from patients who experienced similar episodes of depression. If the patient talks about suicide, you might use such clinical experiences to give the patient hope or to stop them from making a decision they will regret. In either case, formalize the diagnosis by talking about what you are physically seeing and tell them that the symptom matches the diagnosis.

## Step 3

**Be prepared to treat the problem.** If the patient is contemplating suicide, discuss the uncertainty in their life before making a psychiatric referral. Tell the patient that in survivorship, it is common to shuttle back and forth between hope and despair. Since you are not a psychiatrist, resist the impulse to prognosticate the future. Instead, use empathic statements during your conversation about the uncertainty the patient feels and allow them to explore the unpleasantness of the feeling.

Research shows that displacement behaviors can positively align the patient back toward increased participation in the decision-making process and reintegration with life. Near the end of your discussion, consider suggesting a displacement behavior to fill the patient's time. A displacement behavior may take the form of a hobby, an artistic creation, or an intellectual endeavor such as research or education. If the patient shows fear or uncertainty, suggest that the patient research clinical trials or new advances in medicine as a positive displacement behavior. If the patient feels they have nobody to express their fears to, suggest making an artistic creation as a form of that expression. If you suggest a displacement behavior, it is better to suggest one that re-orients the patient to the goals of managed care rather than as a diversion to managed care. If the patient begins to use displacement as a diversion, the behavior may become maladaptive. For this reason, you should monitor the displacement behavior at various points in survivorship.

## CASE STUDY

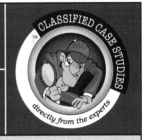

Name: Dr. Scott Sheren
Title: Ophthalmologist
State: New York

The principals of informed consent and patient autonomy both govern my approach to the discussion of treatment options with patients. My clinical experience is of great value in the following regard. I have twenty-six years and more than 10,000 hours of operating room experience, and I have learned that the physician needs to show respect for patient autonomy, which includes individual, physical, emotional, and spiritual needs. The decision-making process is a two-way street. I do not believe that it is possible to have a patient make good decisions about their management plan without having meaningful clear dialogue about the facts of their case, described in language that they can understand. A physician's energy, attitude, and confidence level significantly influences how they retain and process the information presented to them.

I find that when I provide the patient with information, it is helpful to pause frequently so the patient can digest the information, reflect on what I have said, and ask questions based on the information provided. I try to remain open and sensitive to these questions, clarifying and re-interpreting their concerns if I need to, so they can reflect until they summarize the options and contrast the implications of each treatment and arrive at the treatment plan that they believe is best for them. I will argue against the one they have chosen to assure that there is no misunderstanding on their part.

Patient recall tends to diminish during this process due to ongoing fears about the future, and they sometimes will transfer the decision to me. I try to bring this into their awareness so they understand what they are doing. When it comes to elective surgery, I may broach a conversation about emotional readiness because I want them emotionally aligned with the treatment plan, which I believe is particularly important before undergoing invasive procedures.

It is my opinion that the current medical environment too often perverts this process. Many in my profession consider informed consent as a medico-legal process with more emphasis on documentation than an essential part of the doctor-patient relationship. For me, it is an essential part of my professional satisfaction alongside obtaining superior clinical outcomes. When it comes to using visual aids, I normally do not use them. However, I may draw on a pad or make lists to illustrate a point as part of the dialogue. When I do this, I include these notes in the chart and make them handy for future reference to ensure patient understanding.

# Chapter 6

# Communication During Conflict

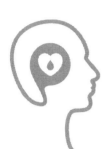

hether you are assisting patients in the decision-making process or breaking bad news
to patients regarding diagnosis or prognosis,
serious medical news is bound to create conflict in most doctor-patient
relationships. When doctors fail to recognize signs of an unfolding conflict, both sides become more frustrated and the clinical relationship
suffers, irreparably in some cases. Conflicts in a medical setting also may
involve conflicts in the relationship between the patient and the family
or conflicts between the physician and the family. Potential conflicts that
commonly arise may include disagreement over treatment, disagreement over disclosure, or relationship conflicts that existed long before
your involvement with the patient's care. This is why early detection

of conflicts can reduce the potential for escalation later on. In order to recognize the signs of conflict, begin with an examination of your own judgments. If you find your frustration level rising, and you begin making negative judgments about the other party, such as labeling them as "clueless" as an excuse to withdraw from the situation, stop yourself from making an emotional, impulsive, or defensive response, and listen to the other person. The ability to do this requires separating your ego from the conflict and asking yourself why the other party opposes another point of view. Since dismissing opposition is the fastest way to get another party to stop listening, you must allow them to voice opposition and acknowledge their view, not just with words but nonverbal communication. If your body language contradicts your words, people will realize that you are simply humoring them.

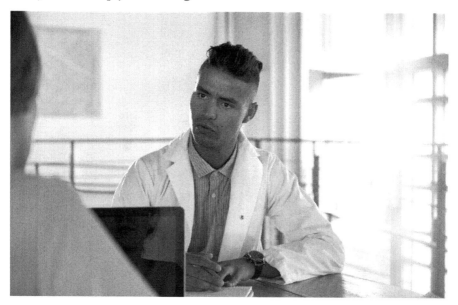

# Types of Conflict

Conflict management requires the use of communication skills that include facilitation, negotiation, and understanding of multiple perspectives. The most common conflict that arises between patients and physicians are those surrounding decisions that one party may consider futile. When only one party considers a decision futile, a conflict may arise over issues of understanding, values, and goals. Decisions surrounding treatment adherence and treatment withdrawal are two common types of futility conflicts that exist between patients and physicians. When your patient sees treatment as futile, they may refuse to comply with treatment adherence. Conversely, you may view some treatments as inappropriate or not beneficial to the patient's management plan whereas the patient believes in the treatment. Researchers refer to this type of frustration as "role conflict." Physicians who feel forced to provide what they believe to be ill-advised medical care out of respect for patient autonomy may experience a conflict with their self-perceived role as a medical expert. Both patients and physicians may feel disrespected if they believe their respective interests go unconsidered by one another. Without properly using communication skills of facilitation, negotiation, and understanding, a clash in feelings and perspectives may not only disrupt the relationship, but also the treatment plan. Conflicts over treatment decisions are most typical when the treatments have not slowed the patient's decline along the illness trajectory (see Chapter 9 for end-of-life communication on treatments requests). In such cases, both parties may experience frustration. The patient may blame the physician for the treatment recommendation, even if the treatment was a shared decision and agreed upon as the best available option. The physician may see the patient's blame as a professional affront without recognizing it as a purely emotional reaction.

Disagreements over disclosure also create conflict between patients and physicians. These types of conflicts are common when the physician wants to disclose information to a third party, but the patient will not allow it. Parents, for example, may feel that disclosing their illness to a child may cause too much distress. Health care practitioners call this behavior "shielding" (when patients want to withhold their medical information from loved ones in order to protect them). However, if the prognosis is terminal, the physician knows they must inform the relatives at some point, and that withholding information may cause greater harm down the road. In this case, the physician may feel frustration over what he or she believes is either selfish behavior or denial. In rare cases, the dynamic of counter-transference may complicate your ability to support the patient's decisions, particularly if they involve disagreements over treatment or disclosure. Counter-transference is a term used in psychoanalysis to describe emotions experienced by the physician when the patient reminds you of someone in your personal life or from your past. Physicians who form an emotional attachment to their patient's medical situation experience counter-transference, which can cloud professional judgment or obstruct support for difficult decisions. For example, if your patient has the same illness your father died from, you might subconsciously see the patient as a second chance to save your father. Motivated by this desire, you wind up recommending an experimental therapy considered high risk, high reward; one that you might otherwise never recommend.

Counter-transference may also complicate any relationship conflicts that may exist between patients and their relatives. Since many families harbor relationship conflicts, chances are excellent that any preexisting relationship conflicts will carry over into the clinical encounter. This is particularly true of conflicts that arise within families who have a history of the illness afflicting the patient. If a relationship conflict exists, opposing parties may force you to choose sides. Counter-transference then may cause you to demonstrate bias and thereby alienate one side. If a family has a long history of conflict, stress brought on by a serious medical situation may exacerbate the inter-relational conflict. Counter-transference and respect for patient autonomy are two common causes of conflict between physicians and the patient's family members. As discussed earlier, foreign cultures tend to place emphasis on family-centered care. Here, the patient's family may forbid you from disclosing information to the patient or assuming all the treatment decisions. Without proper understand of foreign customs and their unique approach to managed care, you may find yourself in conflict with these wishes, particularly if counter-transference plays a role.

Some conflicts do not involve patients or families, but rather, with colleagues or other health care professionals. Conflicts with colleagues can result from disagreements about patient care. Health care practitioners will experience this type of conflict when medical staffers higher in the chain of command give direct orders, which the practitioner is required to obey but disagrees with. For example, nurses may receive orders from physicians not to inform the patient of their diagnosis. Since information sharing is the cornerstone of an effective interdisciplinary team, mistakes in medical care will lead to conflict, especially if a failure in communication channels causes the mistake. For this reason, researchers define the characteristics of a well-functioning team as having clear goals, good leadership, well-defined roles, regular patterns of communication, good record-taking practices, cohesion among team members, established outlets for relieving stress, and mutual respect.

Since emotional involvement in conflict is likely to cloud your judgment and reduce your ability to make good decisions, you must first stop the conflict from escalating. The greater the conflict, the more necessary it becomes to adhere to the basic rules of interviewing. In order to cope with the conflicts described, remain calm, avoid the initial impulse to react, try to take a step back, and use your clinical judgment to decide if the conflict is fixable. If you are able to take a step back, you must define the emotional state of all parties, including yourself. To determine if the conflict is fixable, ask yourself:

- What are my emotions in this conflict?
- How are they influencing the conflict?

- Is it possible for both parties to see the other's point of view?
- Does the opposing party have insight into the way their behavior may be worsening the conflict?
- Is there anything that might motivate either party to change?
- What steps would be required to help them modify their behavior?
- What steps would be required for me to change?

If you answer "no" to these questions, then the problem is unfixable, and your best option to avoid conflict would be to support the patient when deferring to the patient-centered approach, or to the family when deferring to the family-centered approach. If you answer "yes" to these questions, then the problem is fixable. If so, you should then implement communication skills that include facilitation, negotiation, and understanding of multiple perspectives as a way to achieve a mutual definition of the area of conflict. Once you have explored your own emotions, you might begin by describing them (without displaying them) to the opposing party. Sometimes emotions are the direct cause of the conflict rather than the conflict itself, so if you describe your emotions, this may serve as an immediate form of resolution. If the conflict merits further exploration into negotiation, listen to the patient's reasoning, and then try to offer some type of alternative solution, such as referring them to a second opinion or independent broker (as mentioned in Chapter 3). For patients and families, a second opinion may be another doctor, psychiatrist, counselor, or other health care professional. A second opinion allows the opposing party the chance to corroborate or refute your position. While it may seem like questioning of your judgment, you are playing the important role of facilitator to help the patient achieve perspective on the conflict. It is also a means of taking the necessary steps required for one or more parties to change in order to resolve the conflict. If you do decide to offer a second opinion, do not allow the opposing party to push you far from what you believe to be true, especially if you trust your clinical assessment of the conflict. Your purpose in approaching conflict is to provide options available in response to an impasse.

# Signs of Conflict

The best way to manage conflict is to prevent it. So how can you recognize the signs of conflict brewing? Nonverbal signs such as clenched fists, furrowed brows, wringing of the hands, or restricted breathing patterns may indicate the presence of an emotional trigger waiting to escalate. Some patients may indicate conflicts verbally by volunteering buried statements that may hint toward conflicts below the surface of things. For example, if a patient whose cancer is in remission says, "*Sorry if I seem agitated; my husband made me schedule this appointment,*" then the buried statement may indicate a family conflict over the patient's denial and treatment adherence, or perhaps it has nothing to do with the consultation at all. Another patient, in pain and waiting for an hour while you attended to an emergency might quip, "*My time is as valuable as yours, you know.*" In this case, the patient may be expressing misplaced frustration over their pain as anger directed at your absence. Whichever the case, you will never know the underlying causes of conflict unless you acknowledge potential signs of conflict with open questions that elicit invitations to self-expression. Since two of the aforementioned characteristics of a well-functioning medical staff include regular patterns of communication and cohesion among team members, train your medical staff to communicate detection of any warning signs of potential conflict brewing within doctor-patient or patient-family relationships.

Angry, frightened, and defensive patients are the most likely facilitators of conflict, usually geared toward specific entities such as medical staff, their own family, themselves, problems outside their condition, or geared toward abstractions such as their sense of powerlessness or loss of potential. Signs of conflict demonstrated by angry patients include manipulative behaviors, such as issuing threats about suicide or legal action against the hospital. According to Sharon K. Hull and Karen Broquet, "[These types of patients] tend to exhibit impulsive behavior directed at obtaining what they want, and it is often difficult to distinguish between borderline personality disorder and manipulative behavior." Physicians who encounter manipulative patients often expose themselves to the dangers of seduction. These patients may inwardly harbor fear and anger, but outwardly appear nice as a way of controlling the physician's clinical power. Signs of seduction may include sexual seduction, gifts, excessive praise, and increased expectations. If the patient looks to curry special favor and you provide it, it may raise their expectations and legitimize their perceived right to blame you later if those expectations go unfulfilled. In order to manage encounters with manipulative patients, you must:

- Be aware of your own emotions
- Recognize the signs of manipulative behavior
- Attempt to ground the patient's expectations
- Realize that sometimes you have to say no

In most cases, threats serve as defensive mechanisms by which the patient can demonstrate some level of control over what is happening to them. Insecurity and hostility over loss of control are the emotional triggers, and if you let their emotional triggers awaken your own, you will escalate the conflict.

To deal with an angry patient, you can use the nine-step approach to anger outlined in Chapter 3, or respond to the threat by staying calm, identifying and acknowledging the objective of the threat, and asking that the patient suspend the threat. For example, if the patient threatens to stop treatment, you might respond with, "*I find it very difficult to talk about this conflict while you are threatening to stop treatment. Why don't we discuss how you feel, and then, if you still wish to discontinue treatment, we can discuss your right to do so.*" Ensuing discussions may help avoid such rash decisions (such as nonadherence to treatment) by the time you have unearthed the causes of conflict. If the patient issues a suicidal threat, you might respond using closed question as a way to begin removing the threat, such as, "*I know you're depressed, but can we first talk about why you're feeling so desperate?*" This closed statement incorporates an empathic response but goes further because it implies a promise that you will return to the problem they demand you address.

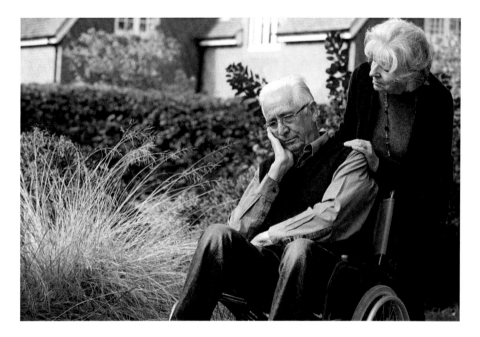

Some signs of conflict arise from some patients who "somatize" their illness and force their doctors into ordering cycles of vigorous diagnostic testing and referrals. According to Hull and Broquet, "These patients present multiple vague or exaggerated symptoms and often suffer from comorbid anxiety, depression, and personality disorders. They often have 'doctor-shopped' and likely have a history of multiple diagnostic tests.

Keys to productive encounters with somatizing patients include describing the patient's diagnosis with compassion and emphasizing that regularly scheduled visits with a primary physician will help to mitigate any concerns." Hull and Broquet also suggest management of comorbid psychological conditions and refraining from telling the patient, "It's all in your head." Other signs of conflict may become manifest through grief. To recognize the signs of conflict brought on by grief, use the Kubler-Ross model to determine if the grief is adaptive or maladaptive. Last, there are patients with enormous medical records who become "frequent fliers" of hospitals. Frequent fliers may exhibit signs of conflict when they base decisions upon records so enormous that they confuse the patient's understanding. In such instances, the physician should provide clarification to avoid conflict. Figure 10 summarizes the components of the difficult clinical encounter.

*Figure 10: Components of a Difficult Clinical Encounter*

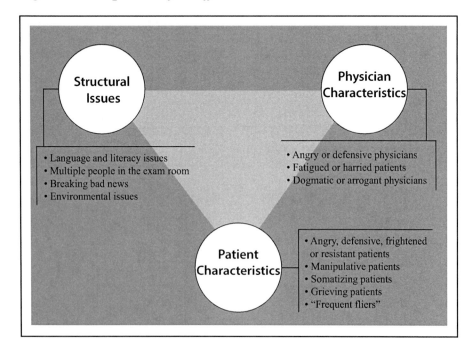

# Road Map to Dealing with Conflict

Physicians can get burned out like anyone else under stress for a prolonged period in their professional life. Dealing with an individual conflict can take its toll on your mental well-being. If you multiply one conflict times a hundred other cases, you might burn out early when the world needs more good doctors like you. The following road map suggested by Anthony Back, Robert Arnold, and James Tulsky in their book, *Mastering Communication with Seriously Ill Patients*, is not for helping patients find their way through stress, but helping you find your way through stress. When you find yourself at odds with someone in your profession, follow this seven-step protocol.

## Step 1

**Identify the conflict.** The conflict may manifest itself as a disagreement, dispute, or difference of opinion. The conflict may involve a patient, a family member, another health professional, or multiple parties. Earlier, we advised that staying calm is the first step in dealing with threats. However, just because you remain calm does not mean the conflict will abate. Conflict may shape itself in other forms, through sarcasm, repeated requests, or passive-aggressive body language.

## Step 2

**Find a nonjudgmental starting point.** The purpose here is to reestablish a dialogue by reframing what you want to discuss in a softer tone. For example, instead of saying, *"You aren't qualified to make a judgment on the best treatment,"* you might reframe the topic regarding qualification and treatments by saying, *"I feel like the treatments I've recommended are the best for you, but if you want* *to hear about other treatments after I've explained why, we can talk about the other treatments. Okay?"*

## Step 3

**Listen to the other person's point of view.** Forget about how you want to respond when the other person speaks. Really listen; do not just wait for your turn to speak because you will not really hear or empathize with their point of view, and they will not feel heard.

## Step 4

**Identify what the conflict is really about and try to identify a shared perspective within the conflict.** Talk about your concerns and keep the focus on the problem, not the people involved in the conflict. Shift the focus of the conflict from blame to best interests.

## Step 5

**Try to brainstorm possible alternative solutions.** Reaching out will, at the very least, show the other party that you have made an honest attempt to address their concerns. This will make it harder for the opposing party to resist your point of view. While you are devising alternatives, do not express your preference; simply explain how they might offer a resolution.

## Step 6

**Brainstorm options that reasonably satisfy all parties involved, or at least recognize their best interests.** Keep in mind that "best interests" is a relative term because the best alternative might be a middling solution for the patient's medical care.

## Step 7

**Realize that not all conflicts can be resolved.** Sometimes you have to say no. If the patient continues to resist, seek a third party to moderate discussion or offer a referral.

# How to Stop Conflicts from Escalating

Robert Buckman's HARD strategy is another road map for dealing with conflict escalation. In an escalating conflict with another person, the limbic system, which controls rage, activates more quickly than the cognitive functions of the neocortex. Because our cognitive functions are slower to activate, irrational anger consumes us, and the result is that we are likely to say or do something we may later regret. According to Buckman, cognitive functions and emotional impulses activate about six seconds apart. During a high emotional exchange, a lot can happen in six seconds. In other words, by the time cognitive functions have begun to activate, your conflict may have escalated to a point of no return. The key to avoiding that first impulse is to wait roughly six seconds before you respond to a patient, family member, or other professional who would escalate a conflict through blame, threats, manipulation or some other means. The HARD strategy is a four-step acronym, **H**igh emotions, **A**cknowledgment, **R**ules, **D**e-escalation.

To know how to de-escalate a conflict, you first have to know something about the nature of conflict escalation. The first step is to recognize the onset of somatic symptoms of high emotions, such as rage. How does your body react to distress? Develop an awareness of somatic symptoms such as increasing pulse rate, an upset stomach, or blood rushing to your head. This also requires personal examination of your psychological triggers. Are you someone who takes things too personally? Do you hate having your authority questioned? Do you sometimes let personal problems affect your professional routine? Knowing how your body and mind reacts to conflict may help you stay rational during those crucial six seconds when you feel the impulse to lash out. Once you let the impulse pass, acknowledge the conflict by admitting to yourself that the situation is getting difficult, and then verbalize it to the other party. You might say something like, "I think this is becoming a difficult situation for both of us." Once you have verbalized the situation, adopt a neutral tone of voice. Tell the other party that you would like to establish rules and boundaries by explaining what you believe is acceptable and what you believe is unacceptable. In any conflict, one person simply may be reacting to another person's demeanor. Body language experts call this type of copycat behavior "mirroring." In such cases, if you allow the person to copy positive body language, that may signal the end of the conflict without further disagreement. If compromise is still necessary, you should de-escalate the situation by suggesting a middle road that each side does not oppose, even if it is not what each side wanted. The important part of de-escalation is to suggest an alternative path that you consider acceptable. It also buys some time, which allows the other party's cognitive functions to return as the limbic system's irrational activation simmers. However — to reiterate the suggestions put forth by Hull and Broquet — if the other party's demands are so unreasonable, there will be times when you just have to say "no." The challenge is to be flexible without compromising your integrity. So, when a conflict appears unresolvable, ask yourself the following questions:

- How important are the other person's core beliefs?
- How important is this to my own core beliefs?

- How flexible can I be in this instance without compromising an important belief of my own?
- What aspects of my identity might feel threatened?
- What might I be denying or exaggerating?
- To what extent am I holding myself to an impossibly perfect standard?
- How can I regain perspective?

If you find that you can be flexible without compromising your important beliefs, you may find yourself more willing to accept what the patient wants and become less attached to biomedical outcomes. If you are not sure that you can be flexible, it may help to seek the guidance of an ethics consultant, palliative care consultant, or colleague.

# Considerations for Nurses

Studies show that a significant percentage of patients with serious diseases such as cancer develop psychiatric and adjustment disorders that lead to conflicts in managed care. Nurses who develop long-term relationships in oncological settings with their patients must be able to recognize (without any psychosocial training) the early warning signs of psychiatric and adjustment disorders. When nurses face the conundrum of choosing between upsetting the patient and addressing the issue, they usually will opt to do nothing out of fear of believing it may harm the patient. In an ambulatory setting, nurses will focus only on the physical aspects of treatment and management of side effects. If the nurse does nothing to address the psychosocial concerns, the problem either will abate or worsen toward some type of conflict. So how do you differentiate between a passing bout of sadness and sadness that needs serious treatment? The medical profession does not expect their nurses to diagnose a major depressive episode, but knowledge of the DSM-IV criteria will help recognize possible symptoms to notify doctors about. Major depressive episodes are not brief. Rather, they tend to manifest over a period. If depressive symptoms and a change in functioning persist over a two-week period, the patient may require treatment.

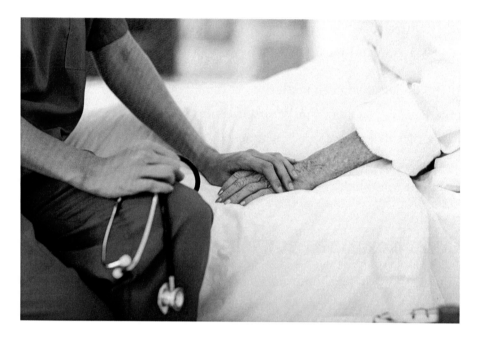

To determine if a doctor should be notified, observe the patient over a two-week period, and run down the criteria listed in DSM-IV, starting with the most common symptoms and working your way down to the least common symptoms. Uncontrolled pain is the most common symptom of a major depressive episode. If the symptoms are not severe, assure the patient that you will treat the problem if the symptoms do not abate over a two-week period. Surprisingly, health professionals report anti-depressants as underutilized in serious medical scenarios because they tend to consider depression as normal and expected. If the patient begins reporting uncontrolled pain, examine the side effects of the treatments administered and determine if they are typical or atypical of the treatment. For example, anti-cancer treatments, in particular, cause side effects resulting from endocrine and metabolic abnormalities, such as euphoria or irritability, which lead to depression. If the treatments are not causing side effects, try to pin down when the uncontrolled pain started, along with the beginning of the symptoms. Risk factors associated with the disease (not the treatment), such as stage advancement, may be causing the uncontrolled pain. Since major depressive episodes also are commonly associated with poorer medical outcomes and decreased quality of life, run a comparative analysis of the patient's medical outcomes and quality of life before the symptoms and after the symptoms. If you do not find evidence of depression caused by treatment or by advancement of disease, obtain the patient's previous medical history and look for signs that might indicate a history of socially induced depression. Signs of socially induced depression might include a reported history of substance use (illegal or prescribed), treatment for anxiety or psychotic disorder, trauma, or bereavement.

To anticipate the possibility of a major depressive episode before one occurs, consider the risk factors associated with depression. Are there statistics that correlate a high incidence of depression with the treatment administered to the patient? Does the patient have an established psychiatric history that might indicate the likelihood of a major depressive episode? Are there social factors that might increase the chances of the patient experiencing depression? If the patient openly talks about suicide, do not ignore it. Instead, invite the patient to discuss what he or she is feeling, as you may uncover a social risk factor not covered in their medical report. However, if you are not prepared to broach the issue, you should have the patient put under watch while you notify a doctor who can make a psychiatric referral. Should you decide to have this discussion, experts recommend that you master key communication skills and process tasks.

To begin a discussion on depression, the nurse should initiate a dialogue that shifts the conversation away from physiological symptoms, such as uncontrolled pain, to emotional concerns, such as their current life stressors. Process tasks for initiating this discussion include creating a setting for privacy, making sure that you are sitting at eye level with the patient, and having tissues at hand. Communication skills required to initiate the discussion may include making a statement that acknowledges a change in behavior, asking open-ended questions, and normalizing the patient's feelings so they understand that their feelings are justified and common. Shifting from physiological to emotional concerns allows the nurse to assess the patient's needs and provides an opportunity for them to educate the patient about depression.

During your discussion with the patient, ask direct questions about the patient's emotional distress. According to a 2003 study published by the *American Journal of Psychiatry* on the assessment and practice guidelines for patients with suicidal behaviors, patients are more likely to reveal the true nature of their distress when nurses approach these concerns with self-confidence. Process tasks for responding to these distresses may include validating the distress as reasonable, and praising their attempts to cope with the distress. If the patient says something you do not understand, ask for clarification of the intended meaning. When the patient clarifies, you might restate the explanation as a way of checking for your own understanding. At the end of the discussion, summarize and review the patient's emotional experience and try to connect them to one of the risk factors so the patient can gain some clarity on cause and effect. Afterward, use the process task of exploring the patient's attitude about possible treatment for depression. The communication skills necessary to complete this task include expressing your willingness to help, making a statement about being available to help the patient decide, going over the steps required to initiate treatment for depression, inviting questions, and offering the patient time to think about the option.

# Considerations for Social Workers

When doctors and nurses in palliative or hospice care settings find themselves unable to explore or resolve issues beyond biomedical outcomes, they may consider bringing in a social worker to reduce conflicts of psychosocial concern. Social work is about promoting social change and solving problems in human relationships. In the medical setting, social work has a long history with helping seriously ill patients and their families. Whether you are a doctor adhering to the rules of patient autonomy or a social worker promoting human rights, your objective is the same: you must find a way to help the patient through a time of conflict and crisis. If you are a social worker assigned to a seriously ill patient, you must find out what has brought about crisis in the patient's life by examining your case in three aspects: context, situation, and meaning.

Context refers to the factors that make the patient's situation unique from other situations you have encountered. The uniqueness of the patient's conflict may involve one or a combination of factors, which may include age, gender, social history, relationships, previous life-altering experiences, current level of social support, cultural background, and economic status. Social workers typically examine two contexts when trying to understand the individual's conflicts. The first context involves the unique characteristics that shaped them; the second context is relational (i.e. the individual in relation to others, such as family and friends). Examination of relational context matters more when the conflict presents itself relationally, whether between family members or other members of society. Relational context also matters more in cultures that use a family-centered approach to managed care, and this is where individual and relational contexts overlap.

After gaining an understanding of individual and relational context, examine the situation that created the conflict. To begin your analysis of the current situation, get a first-hand account of the crisis from everyone involved in the crisis, and use the accounts to trace the events leading up to the crisis back to its transition point. The transition point is the triggering event that moved the situation from static to conflict. For example, let us suppose you encounter a patient who, upon examining the individual and relational context of the situation, appeared to cope well with their initial diagnosis. Then, after speaking with each member involved in the conflict, you discover that the patient stopped coping well when an estranged relative came to visit the patient. You might conclude that the transition point occurred when the estranged relative arrived. However, you dig a little further and discover that the arrival of the estranged relative coincided with the patient's cancer recurrence. Did the transition point occur because the relative showed up or because the cancer came out of remission? Upon further examination, you discover that the patient's cancer recurrence may have triggered relational issues with the estranged relative. You then explore the relationship between the two possible trigger events. You discover that the same disease the patient suffers from physically debilitated the estranged relative. You then go back to the patient's psychosocial history and learn that the patient makes a living at something that requires physical coordination. In this scenario, you might conclude that the presenting problem (the disease and the relative) was not the cause of the crisis, and that the underlying problem (fear of losing economic potential) served as a transition point into conflict.

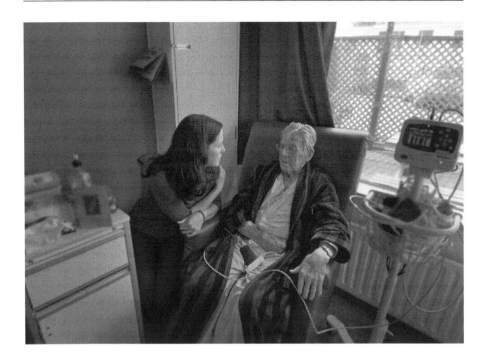

Once you have identified the transition point and underlying problem, you must work to bring the person from a state of distress and conflict to a state of coping and resolution. While the underlying problems may create conflict, you must examine and address the conflict as viewed through the eyes of the patient. Therefore, you must ask, what type of meaning does this conflict have for the patient? If other parties involved in the conflict do not view the situation as a conflict, communicate the patient's perspective to the opposing party so that they can begin to understand why the conflict has caused the patient distress. To implement a strategy of communication, ascertain the patient's safety by ruling out potential issues that might endanger the patient. If the psychosocial history does not provide indicators of imminent physical or mental danger, assess the crisis by asking questions designed to gain information, to check for understanding, and to test your theories about the situation.

When you assess the underlying cause and transition point, stage a conflict intervention by breaking down the issue into smaller crises and dealing with each of them separately. Using the previous example, you might break down the issue of the patient's cancer recurrence as a separate issue from relationship conflict with the estranged relative. It some cases, you will find it necessary to further break down the context, situation, and meaning of the conflict by relational value. For example, instead of limiting your examination of the patient's cancer recurrence through the relational value with the estranged relative, you look at the patient's roles as child, parent, friend, or employee. Using these additional factors you ask, how does each of my client's relational roles influence or change the context, situation, and meaning of the conflict? From there, identify potential barriers for conflict resolution and work to develop strategies that might allow all parties involved to seek resolution.

## CASE STUDY

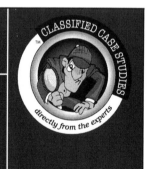

Name: M. Gregg Bloche
Title: Professor of Law
at Georgetown University /
author of The Hippocratic Myth
District: Washington, D.C.

**Excerpt Taken From:** Managing Conflict at the End of Life, **www.nejm.org**

Anger, denial, and other irrational influences can lock family members into warring stances over whether to treat a devastating illness aggressively or discontinue life-sustaining measures. What is remarkable, given the intensity of the feelings at stake, is how rarely such conflicts make their way to court. It is a measure of how discreetly families handle squabbles. To rend families asunder at the end of a loved one's life does spiritual violence to all concerned. Within wide boundaries, we are committed to honoring patients' clearly stated wishes. This commitment not only safeguards patients' liberty and dignity; it protects against family strife when a patient's intentions are clear. When the patient's wishes are unstated and illness precludes asking about them, it is important to limit the possibilities for family conflict and lasting anger. Enabling families to mourn and move on — and discouraging them from playing out old resentments as end-of-life battles — should be a clinical and social priority.

When conflict erupts, physicians should not treat end-of-life choices as purely ethical questions, divorced from the regrets and resentments involved. Psychiatric and social work consultation should be part of the management plan, and mediation merits study as an approach. Communication methods that foster listening, exploring needs, reframing problems, and proposing solutions help guide warring family members toward agreement on end-of-life choices for their loved one.

At times, physicians, and even insurers, become parties to these conflicts. Financial incentives, real or perceived, can shape positions and sow distrust. Cost-control strategies that engage caregivers in covert rationing can have toxic effects, particularly when medical futility is at issue. Our national unwillingness to acknowledge the conflict between efforts to limit medical spending and insistence on all possibly beneficial care worsens this toxicity. Good mediation technique can help to clarify misunderstandings, soften anger, and ease irrational distrust.

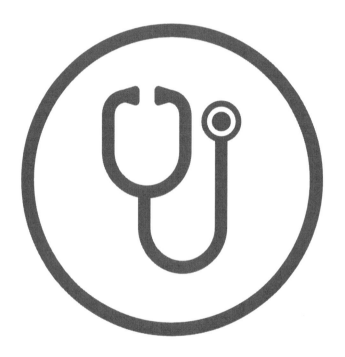

# Chapter 7

# Communicating with the Patient's Family

ommunicating with members of the patient's family may require using some of the previously discussed guidelines in order to discuss negative medical news, particularly when it comes to dealing with local conflicts. Local conflicts may occur when priorities of the family conflict with the patient's autonomy. For example, in Chapter 6, we discussed the concept of "shielding," which occurs when patients want to withhold their medical information from loved ones in order to protect them. Conversely, when family members are the first to discover the patient's medical situation, they may ask that you withhold medical information from the patient in order to protect their loved one. Shielding a patient who may lack autonomy (such as a child or advanced elder) is easier than shielding a patient who understands the situation and has the right to make informed choices. When priorities clash between family members and patients with a clear right to autonomy, the patient's priorities take precedence.

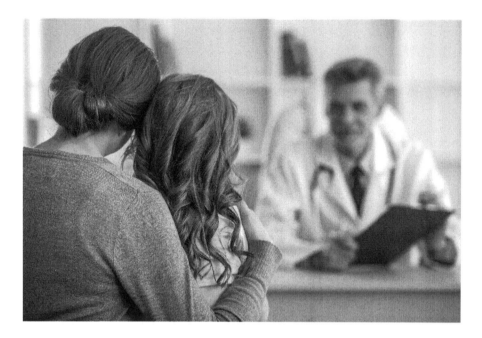

In any local conflict, you must honor the patient's autonomy despite the family's wishes, but still seek to identify and acknowledge the feelings and perspectives of the family. Performing the latter requires communication skills aimed at dealing with the family's priorities in some way, especially if the patient's choices have direct consequences on the lives of the family. For example, when the patient becomes sick, the family members may inherit the role of primary caregiver. Family members who become the primary caregiver therefore have a vested personal interest in the health management plan. Let us suppose you consult with a patient who wants to try a promising but potentially risky phase I clinical trial. After making the patient aware of the trial status, the patient decides to enroll. With the patient's permission, you inform the family of the decision and the family protests the decision due to the inherent risks that may increase their burden as caregiver. If the patient's priority is to get well at any cost, and the family's priority is to minimize their burden, here you have the genesis of local conflict. The family will lobby for the standard treatment options while the patient elects to go with the high risk, high reward solution. Oftentimes, the key to resolving a local conflict means trying to find a solution that satisfies the priorities of both the patient and the family. Arranging a family meeting will be your best means of providing support.

# The Role of the Family in a Clinical Encounter

Regardless of whether a conflict between the patient and the family arises, you will have to arrange a family meeting shortly after making a diagnosis — and possibly several other meetings afterward. The first family meeting should orient the patient and the family to the disease, review treatment options, and provide an overview of all support channels. The next family meeting may occur in the midst of ongoing therapy to review the results of therapy and possibly redefine the goals of managed care. If your patient is in palliative care, you should hold a family meeting to plan ongoing managed care. If a local conflict arises over the goals of care, the purpose of your family meeting should focus on the disagreement as it relates to the clinical objective. To avoid a potential conflict of interest that may develop further down the line, the first family meeting after the diagnosis may include:

- Clinical education about the illness
- Assessment of the caregivers' needs
- Electing a liaison to the medical team
- Plans for unexpected scenarios
- Identifying the decision maker(s)

- Discussions about the next steps
- Assessment of family risk factors
- Possible referrals

Assessing family risk factors may influence how you handle the other goals outlined above. For example, if you identify a family as high risk for local conflicts, you may have to remediate differences as they relate to education, caregiving, decision-making, unexpected scenarios, and future plans. Making determinations as to whether families are at increased risk of local conflicts requires exploration of critical family functions, such as cohesion between members, their economic capacity, their social values, and their protectiveness of one another. Families that demonstrate high function in all four categories are at lower risk of local conflict than families who demonstrate poor function. High-functioning families demonstrate protective behaviors that put the needs of the sick family member first, have the economic means to meet their caregiving respon-sibilities, demonstrate the ability to resolve their squabbles by reorganiz-ing their roles and priorities, and demonstrate strong values through constructive engagement and adherence to social norms. Dysfunctional families demonstrate combativeness amongst each other, reject support, cling to their individual priorities, exhibit signs of depression, or express worries about providing basic means of economic support.

Due to the advances in medicine, the role of the family as caregiver has increased along with the number of patients now receiving therapy from home. Recent studies show that spouses are the primary caregivers in roughly 70 percent of home care settings. Children comprise 20 percent while distant relatives comprise the remaining 10 percent. When dis-cussing the caregiver's role in the first family meeting, it is important to discuss the responsibilities that come with symptom management, such as educating the caregiver about medications, when to seek outside help, and how to seek outside help. To prepare the caregiver for the responsibilities that lie ahead, accentuate the positive aspects of caregiving when talking about the emotional demands of the role. Often, this means brainstorming sources of additional support from volunteers or community resources. The main goal of the initial family meeting and subsequent meetings is to facilitate and promote movement toward group consensus. Therefore, you should partition the family meeting into two parts: the clinical encounter and the psychosocial encounter. The clinical encounter covers the medical aspects of the illness, including the illness trajectory, list of available treatments with their risks and benefits, protocols for medical management, and future treatment options. The psychosocial encounter covers the emotional and potential lifestyle impact of the illness on the family, aspects of coping, and the range of family needs.

The range of family needs may be clinical or psychosocial in nature. Clinical needs include education on how to administer treatments, how to ambulate, how to prepare meals, and how to coordinate visits from support services. Psychosocial needs may include practices for minimizing or overcoming burnout and exhaustion. The family meeting offers an opportunity to introduce the family to the medical staff. When you arrange a family meeting, identify who will attend, which relatives are the most influential, and which medical staffers should be present to provide assistance to your clinical or psychosocial discussions. Once you have set up the meeting, seek input from the family to determine if the medical agenda you have laid out conflicts with any psychosocial needs. During the meeting, determine their strengths and vulnerabilities, and familiarize them with resources designed to address these points. Resources may include educational materials, DVDs, websites, or any of the decision-making aids outlined in Chapter 5.

# The Convergence Model of Communication

In the early stages of communication research, linear models of communication dominated the landscape of practical application. In linear models, information between doctor and patient flows one way, and since paternalistic relationships with patients were the accepted practice of the times, it made sense that no other type of model emerged until 1979 when D. Lawrence Kincaid proposed a new model in Pater 18 of the *East-West Communication Institute Monograph*. The convergence model of communication became the first non-linear model of communication designed to achieve mutual understanding between two or more communicators through multidirectional information flow. Kincaid justified the elimination of linear communication by identifying problems that existed in the established western models, which often led to breakdowns in communication or undesirable results. The problems Kincaid cited in linear models included message source biases, lack of attention to larger contexts, overemphasis on persuasion, and casual neglect of understanding, relationships, and mutual causation. Under Kincaid's new model, communication strategies should push differing emotions, opinions, and priorities into a convergence area of mutual agreement. Communication strategies in the convergence model do not require gaining total acceptance by opposing parties, but rather a pursuit of a common ground, leaving open areas of non-convergence where opinions and priorities remain in misunderstanding and disagreement.

Similar to Degner's spectrum of decision-making models, the convergence model shown in Figure 11 forms an overlap (or common ground) between dyads and triads. A dyadic convergence is an alternate solution that forges a common ground between two parties. A triadic convergence is an alternate solution that forges a common ground between three parties. In figure 11a, we see the process of convergence unfold as two dyads understand, perceive, and interpret information differently. As communication strategies unfold, both parties reach a convergence area of collective understanding, agreement, and action.

When you have identified families at risk in at least one of the four categories of family function, chances are excellent that you will encounter a number of local conflicts. Thus, your challenge as facilitator will be to overcome the communication barriers created by those who may disrupt the clinical or psychosocial agenda. When dysfunctional families interact, relatives may bog down the process of multidirectional communication by interrupting each other or forcing you to choose sides. In order to maintain the path to convergence, avoid taking sides, acknowledge that different perspectives exist, and firmly control and direct the conversation so everyone has equal speaking time without interruptions.

*Figure 11. Convergence Model of Communication*

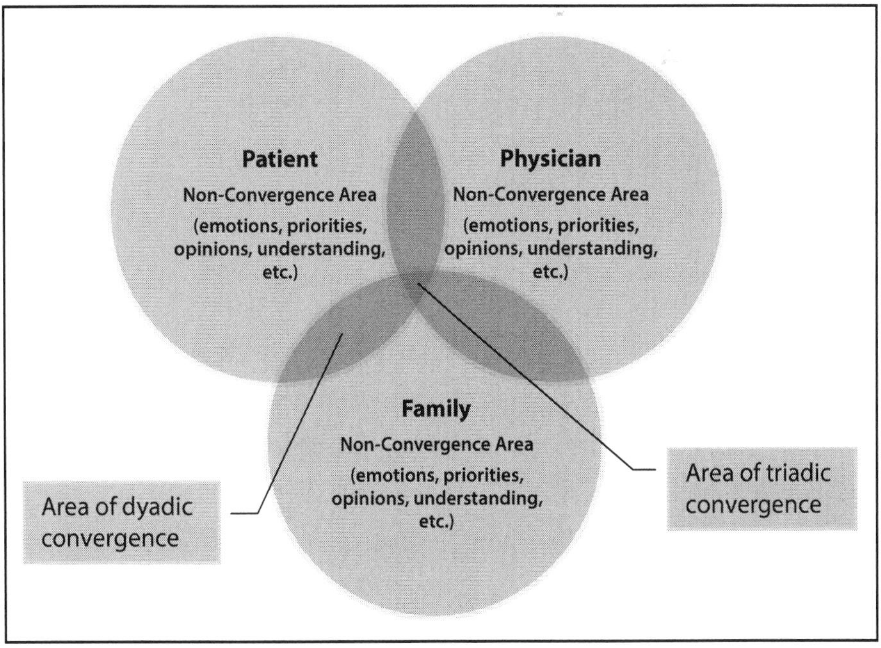

*Figure 11a. The Process of Convergence*

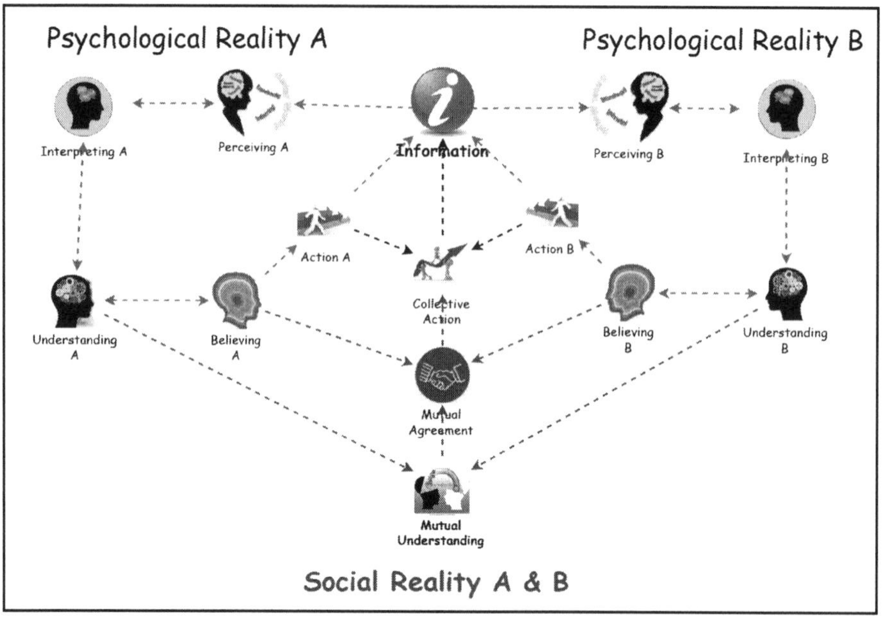

# Conducting a Family Meeting

Before you arrange a family meeting, it is helpful to meet with the patient and ask questions about family dynamics. How does the family make decisions? Do they get along? Who are the relatives with strong personalities? Do they tend to have diverging opinions or high emotions? Have they shown an ability to make compromises in the past? Asking these types of questions will give you a sense of the family's adaptability in the four categories of function so you know if you are dealing with a low-, moderate-, or high-risk family. By doing so, you are laying the groundwork for creating a neutral discussion when the family meeting takes place. Since any meeting between the patient, physician, and family is triadic, start the process of achieving triadic convergence by using a road map. In their book, *Mastering Communication with Seriously Ill Patients*, Anthony Back, Robert Arnold, and James Tulsky offer an eight-step protocol for giving serious news in a family meeting.

## Step 1

**Prepare for the meeting.** Preparations include determining which family members to invite. While this involves the input and permission of the patient, any relative who wishes to partake should be able to attend unless the autonomous patient states otherwise. When choosing which relatives to invite, it is important to appear impartial, or you risk the appearance of taking sides. Upon finalizing the invitation, meet with your medical staff to coordinate the agenda and formulate a clear and consistent message. Choose a private setting to host the meeting.

## Step 2

**Introduce all participants at the meeting and state their purpose for attending.** If members of your medical staff attend, ask them to give their names and their role in caregiving. Afterward, ask the relatives in attendance to state their relationship to the patient and caregiving responsibilities. When introducing yourself to each family member, consider using the techniques of building rapport outlined in Chapter 2. Preview the agenda by telling the family what you would like to discuss, and then ask everyone present if they have any relevant issues they would like to address following your clinical discussion. Here is where you may encounter local conflicts due to non-convergence in understanding, priority, opinion, or emotion. If things get heated, remind the relatives you just want a list of issues, and that you will address each issue in detail later in the meeting. If a relative starts asking questions before you have completed Step 2, promise to answer those questions after introductions.

## Step 3

**Ask the family what it knows about the illness, what they have observed, and what they expect to happen.** Their answers will provide an assessment of their clinical understanding and give you an idea about which perspectives exist in non-convergence. Consequently, their clinical understanding of the situation (or lack thereof) may also hint at emotional and psychosocial data.

## Step 4

**Describe the clinical situation.** Create an overview that lasts no longer than a few minutes. Afterward, check the patient and the family for understanding.

## Step 5

**Ask each member of the family to voice their concerns.** If the family raised concerns or asked premature questions, here is where you fulfill your earlier promise by returning to their concerns. Remember to remain impartial and recognize family members equally, even if you feel one relative is being cruel or unfair. In many cases, this kind of behavior predates the illness and reflects lifelong patterns of interaction. If you sense the conflict escalating, use the HARD strategy outlined in Chapter 6 to defuse the situation. Remember that since you cannot solve poor communication tactics and lifelong patterns of behavior, your goal throughout this part of the meeting is to keep the focus on the patient's values. If a family relative exhibits cruel or unfair behavior that does not fit a lifelong pattern, the relative is probably expressing anger toward the illness. The classification of family anger includes:

- Anger against the patient (possible cause: the patient's carelessness or the relative's fear of abandonment)

- Anger against other family members (possible cause: the belief that another relative contributed to the cause of the disease)

- Anger against the medical staff or institution (possible cause: blaming the messenger, loss of control, for communication gaps or uncaring doctors)

- Anger against outside forces (possible cause: working conditions that contributed to the cause of the disease)

- Against God (possible cause: fear of spiritual abandonment and a sense of unfairness)

Once the entire family has aired any differences, acknowledge the local conflict by saying something like, "I can see that many of you have disagreements. I wonder if you could put these differences aside for now, so that we can focus on helping [the patient]." You might follow by asking, "Is there anything that I or my staff can do to help you through this difficult time?" If the family demonstrates the ability to put their differences aside, acknowledge this action, as it may help bring the group closer toward convergence. If the family shows no sign of dissension, praise their ability to work collectively and continue to Step 6.

## Step 6

**Explore the patient's values.** The purpose of this step is to demonstrate to the family that the patient's values take precedence and should influence the medical decisions. If the patient is unable physically to make the decisions, you might ask the family members in charge of making the decisions what the patient would do if they were able to. While this may conflict with their own desires, it teaches the family to respect the patient's values and to reconsider any decision that would appear self-serving.

**Step 7**

**Propose the goals of care that put the patient's values first.** Start by talking about applicable therapies. Keep the list short; otherwise, you may invite further dissension and indecision among relatives about which therapy best achieves the desired goals. Be prepared to negotiate the goals of your clinical agenda.

**Step 8**

**Provide a follow-up plan.** Summarize the main points that you want the family to take away from the meeting, and talk about setting milestones for reviewing therapies and clinical decisions. Afterward, thank the family for coming in, and tell them you will arrange future meetings as necessary.

# Sharing Bad News with a Patient's Family

Before you can arrange a meeting and practice the strategies for convergence, you must know the rules of sharing bad news with family members. The first rule is that you must always obtain the patient's consent to share bad news. You can ask before the family meeting when determining attendance or at the beginning of a patient interview while a family member is present. If the patient wishes to discuss information in private during a patient interview, tell the relative that the patient would like to have a private discussion rather than asking the patient to leave. Framing your statement as a patient request lets the relative know that the patient is making the request. Since patient interviews are different from family meetings, the relative will not feel alienated and may be less inclined to challenge the desires of a loved one. If the patient is mentally incompetent, you are required to discuss the condition with the next of kin.

By legal definition, next of kin refers to the spouse, or the nearest blood relatives of the patient, whether it is a parent or child. Next of kin also includes anyone who would inherit part of the patient's estate by the laws of descent and distribution if no will exists. In order to determine next of kin, go back to the medical records where you recorded the family history, look at the family tree, and determine next of kin by the rule of degrees. The rule of degrees will help you determine each relative's distance by blood. For example, a child is one degree removed from the parent; a grandchildren and siblings are two degrees removed, and so on down the line of descendants. All states have statutes that specify the process with minor variations. To determine your state's next of kin laws, contact your state legislature. An online guide is available at **http://thomas.loc.gov/home/state-legislatures.html**.

# Model Statements for Communicating with Families

*The Handbook of Communication in Oncology and Palliative Care* offers model statements for communicating with families of patients facing serious illness. Physicians can use model statements to fulfill their role in the family meeting, which includes validating family members and restating information to help the family achieve convergence. Using model statements helps to engage family members and address the challenges of convergence presented by conflicts in relationships. Table 3 lists the model statements suggested for use in an oncological or palliative care setting.

*Table 3. Strategies and Model Statements for the Family Meeting*

| Strategy | Model Statement |
|---|---|
| When introducing yourself to family members | "I'm Dr...it is good to meet you; I am glad you're here." |
| When you need to identify other important relatives who are not present | "Are there other family members or people close to you that you want to be included, either at the next visit or by a phone call?" |
| When you have to elicit concerns and expectations from relatives | "Do you have any particular questions or concerns that you would like to discuss today?" |
| When you need to check for accuracy | "Am I correct in saying that your question about the patient's condition is...?" |
| When you need to check for agreement | "It's seems that we all think that treatment x looks like it might be a good choice for us to consider.... Does everyone agree?" |
| When you need to initiate convergence | "It's important that we try to reach a common ground about the best treatment choices, so let's talk about how we can get there." |

| Strategy | Model Statement |
|---|---|
| When you need to reassure relatives | "You have every reason to feel helpful and reassured that you're doing everything possible to help." |
| When you need to address a relative's resistance to the patient undergoing experimental treatment options | "It is understandable that you feel this treatment might be risky, but I can assure you that we have looked into its safety and effectiveness based on other patients who have taken it." |
| When you need to control a family member's dominant or interruptive behavior | "I understand how you feel about this. I would like to give everyone equal time to hear their opinions in their own words." |
| When you need to address an angry response to a medical outcome | "These treatments do not always work the way we hope and expect. We are all understandably upset when it happens." |
| When you need to address a relative's denial of test results | "It maybe hard to understand the test results given that [the patient] does not seem to feel sick or show symptoms." |

# Questions that Facilitate Family Meetings

As you engage the patient's family, asking three types of questions can further facilitate the meeting and help you reach your clinical and psychosocial objectives. When you want to promote curiosity and reflection among the group, you ask a circular question. A circular question asks one family member to comment on the perspective of another family member. Circular questions enable relatives to air their differences that they might otherwise keep to themselves. For example, you might ask one relative who they believe to be the most upset in the group, or how well they feel that the person has coped with the situation. Circular questions allow family members to gain new perspectives by "seeing themselves from the outside." When you want to promote brainstorming of possibilities or imagine future outcomes, you ask a reflexive question. Reflexive questions work well for situations where quality of life issues are at stake. For example, you might ask the group if they can come up with positive reasons for why the patient should transition to hospice care. When you want to incorporate your own solution into the wording of a question without actually making the recommendation, you ask a strategic question. A strategic question works well when you want to guide families toward decisions without seeming intrusive. For example, if you think the family needs to discuss changing treatments, you might ask them what negative effects they would have to see in order to think about changing treatments. If they start talking about symptoms, you can use this as a preamble for talking about the symptoms you are seeing in order to broach the issue of changing treatments. If these questions elicit discussions that reveal tensions or differing opinions that exist, highlight these tensions and opinions by summarizing what you have heard. After you break the meeting, document everything that occurred. Your documentation should include:

- Who attended the meeting
- Who did not attend the meeting
- A genogram (names, genders, ages, and relationships within the family)

- A meeting summary outlining the issues addressed and options discussed
- A follow-up plan
- Whether information in the meeting was shared with the patient

# Dealing with Anticipatory Grief and Other Emotions

Earlier in this book, we discussed responding to patients who experience a range of emotions in the Kubler-Ross extended cycle of grief. When receiving serious medical news about loved ones, relatives also may experience the extended grief cycle after learning that the patient has a short amount of time left to live. Relatives of the patient experience what clinicians call "anticipatory grief." Anticipatory grief is the cycle of grieving that occurs before a patient diagnosed with serious illness has died. When family members experience anticipatory grief, reassure them that what they are feeling is a normal and adaptive behavior that can help them prepare for impending loss. It is also an opportune time to talk about the value of bereavement services and recommend a grief counselor.

Some relatives will find anticipatory grief confusing if they do not understand why they grieve before anyone has died. They may confuse it with some other emotion apart from the Kubler-Ross extended grief cycle — namely fear and guilt — if not properly distinguished. Even if the patient has a short time to live, the patient remains your primary responsibility. However, when the patient dies unexpectedly, and you have to break the news to next of kin, the patient's relatives become your primary responsibility. In other words, in your role as physician, the patient's wellness is no longer your concern as a health provider, so your responsibility shifts to supporting the wellness of the living. When relatives learn that their loved one has unexpectedly passed, they may experience remorse over unspoken conversations or unfinished family resolutions. When the relatives become your "patient," encourage them to express what they intended to say. You might model a statement by saying, "If he were here right now, what would you want to say to him?" Research shows that when grieving relatives describe their emotions and verbalize what they would have told their deceased, this can have a healing effect on the relative. When a parent or spouse dies, the relative may express fear for their own future, whether driven by economic concerns or genetic risk of contracting the same illness. Informing family members that their loved one has unexpectedly passed involves several process tasks, which include:

- Finding a special interview room and creating an appropriate physical setting
- Introducing yourself
- Finding out when the family last saw the patient alive
- Finding out if the family were the ones who discovered the patient dead
- Being prepared to confirm the patient's death if the relatives want you to get to the point
- Using empathic statements
- Making sure a bereavement specialist is available to see the family

Finding out when the family last saw the patient alive allows you to anticipate the family's reaction. They may have had some idea that the patient was sick, so exploring what they know about the situation will give you an idea about how shocking the news will seem to them. Next, ask the relatives what they thought about the situation at the time, but do not give them the option of asking what they want to know about the new developments. Instead, give a brief description of what happened. Relatives will be able to digest bad news more easily if you present the events as a narrative. For example, you might say, "The surgery caused complications to his heart, and it stopped beating. We tried to resuscitate him, but we could not revive his heart. I am sorry to tell you that your [relative] has died." Finding out if the family discovered the patient dead means they may have some idea that the patient is seriously injured, but they are not sure about the patient's current condition. This scenario is most common in vehicular accidents where the surviving relative was involved in the accident.

While research shows that patients report greater dissatisfaction with physicians who break bad news over the phone, this practice is more accepted when it comes to informing relatives of serious medical news. If you have to inform a relative that their loved one has died, make sure you are speaking to the right person. In this case, the right person would be next of kin. Next, introduce yourself and speak slowly so the relative has time to become oriented to the nature of the phone call. Make an early point of saying that you would prefer to talk in person, but a phone call is the only way to notify next of kin in these circumstances. Prepare the relative for your declaration by saying that you have bad news. Follow this statement by using a narrative to break the news and offer your condolences. If the relative gives an emotional response, use an empathic statement and ask if the relative has someone who can help them, especially if the relative must come to the hospital to identify the body.

# Communicating Genetic Risk to Families

Communicating information about disease sometimes means communicating genetic risk to family members. Family members of patients who develop specific cancers fall into three categories of genetic risk: high risk, moderate risk, and average risk. High-risk individuals have a number of relatives who developed cancer before the relative you are treating. Moderate-risk individuals have a couple of previously affected relatives, and average-risk individuals have few or no relatives affected. Individuals at high risk may seek consultation from their primary care physician or cancer specialist. If you are the health care practitioner the individual seeks out, your communication of genetic risk will involve conceptualizing probabilities based on quantitative derivations (such as cancer population statistics) to individual risk (such as family history suggesting inheriting genes and mutations in DNA repair). Facilitating a relative's comprehension of risk is critical to their decision about whether to have a genetic test performed. To assist comprehension, present a number of communication formats and ask the relative which they prefer. Most people prefer a communication format of words to numbers because words address uncertainty better than numbers. Whichever format you choose, researchers recommend using concrete, case-based information rather than abstract, statistical information because it personalizes the implications.

When you provide a clinical explanation, stick to providing information about cause, severity, prevention, and treatment options. If you detect misplaced anxiety, address it with the relative. If you are able to identify a cancer predisposing mutation, advise the at-risk relative to test for this mutation. If the patient resists discussing genetic risk with family members, identify the barrier preventing the patient from discussing it. The barrier may be a positive motivation such as "shielding," a negative motivation such as family conflict, or a neutral motivation such as denial that any genetic risk exists. Once you have identified the motivation, use the techniques outlined in this book to elicit a discussion about the motivation. In conjunction to verbal communication about genetic risk, researchers recommend using videotapes, audiotapes, written summaries, and leaflets. Risk communication aids can produce higher comprehension, lower decisional conflict, and more active participation. According to the *Handbook of Communication in Oncology and Palliative Care*, "a combination of verbal and written communication with family members results in more relatives contacting genetic services about their risk than either form of communication alone."

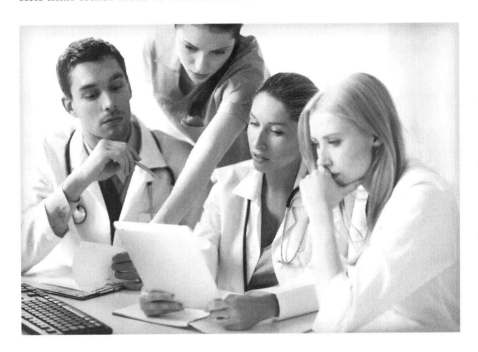

# When Families Make Decisions for Patients

If your patient is unconscious, in a coma, or mentally and physically unable to make decisions for themselves, family members are ethically empowered to become the decision makers. Physicians who handle these cases should inquire if the patient has executed a power-of-attorney for health care. If the patient has executed a power of attorney for health care, there may be an advanced directive that details the patient's medical wishes, including specific details about what treatment is or is not acceptable to them. These legal documents should identify the person entitled to make decisions on behalf of that patient. If no such document exists, you may appoint next-of-kin or someone professionally entitled to make these decisions. If family members become surrogate decision-makers, your role as the health care practitioner is to guide them through the decision-making process as if they were the patient. As a general rule of thumb, if the decisions involve multiple decision-makers, try to use convergence techniques to help them achieve consensus about medical treatment. If they cannot reach unanimous consensus, the majority decision should prevail. If a family member opposes the majority decision, tell them that the law allows physicians to proceed with the majority opinion in cases of multiple surrogate decision-making. Surrogate decision-making also permits the surrogates to decline life-sustaining treatment, if consensus prevails that withdrawal of treatment is in the patient's best interest. If you are unsure about any legal requirements in surrogate decision-making, consult Appendix J, or The Family Health Care Decisions Act, which governs health care decisions for patients who lack autonomy.

# Pitfalls of Surrogate Decision-Making

When no advanced directives exist, communicating with surrogate decision makers comes with certain pitfalls that you would be wise to avoid. The most common pitfall involves asking family members to decide on life-sustaining treatments. Physicians make the mistake of asking, "What do you want us to do?" when they should be using the communication tool of framing the question in a way that asks what the patient would have wanted. Instead, you might say, "If she could talk for herself, what do you think she would she want us to do?" The second pitfall occurs when the health practitioner relies too much on the input of a single, legal surrogate decision maker. If a relative has a power-of-attorney right to make the final decision, you must respect and obey that decision. At the same time, try to use the communication tool of incorporating the input of other family members — even if they fall below the decision-making hierarchy — to achieve a consensus. By doing so, you may also be saving the empowered decision maker the anguish of blaming themselves if they make a decision that has unexpected negative consequences for the patient. If you can reach a consensus agreement, you lessen the burden of decision-making and its consequences, good or bad. This pitfall overlaps into another pitfall — overlooking the burden of caregiving and stress. Studies show that caregiving can carry not only a heavy emotional toll on the caregiver, but also a financial one, which puts them at risk of post-traumatic stress disorder. To help surrogates cope, monitor their coping behavior and look for signs of stress. If you detect maladaptive problems, offer to explore the nature of their stress or provide a support service.

# Dealing with Collusion

Collusion is the act of arranging a secret agreement between two or more people to deceive another person with the purpose of obtaining something they would not be able to achieve through legitimate means. Collusion in the medical setting occurs when professionals agree with relatives to "shield" patients from emotionally harmful information by withholding certain aspects of their medical information. Cultures that take the patient-centered approach to medicine consider this an unethical practice. If the patient's family members are asking you to collude, the following framework will help you manage collusion.

First, it is important to recognize the motivation behind collusion — that high anxiety levels and a need for the relative to protect their loved ones are the cause of most collusion requests. Second, shift your focus from your responsibility to the patient to the person asking you to collude. Third, arrange a private meeting to explore the causes behind their request. During your discussion, make a point of demonstrating how the emotional cost of collusion to the individual, the family, and the patient can be heavier than telling the patient the truth. Consider using examples of stories you have heard about collusion and their detrimental effects. Talk about the questions asked by the patient and suggest to the relative that the patient may already know or will eventually discover the truth regardless of any attempt to hide it. At the end of this discussion, tell the relative that you will interview the patient, and assure the relative that you will only provide the truth if the patient asks or if they appear ready to hear it. Remind the relative that the patient reserves the right to refuse disclosure, and that you are obligated to honor that.

## Talking to Parents of Sick Children

If you have children, then you can imagine the pain experienced by parents of sick children in your care. Talking to parents of sick children can be difficult for some health practitioners, especially when countertransference plays a role. Since children are unable to make autonomous decisions, the parent automatically becomes the legal representative and surrogate decision maker for them. As surrogate and legal representative, the parent's emotional difficulties increase tenfold, as they carry the burden of decision-making and consequence. They inappropriately may feel that the burden of the illness rests squarely on their shoulders. Unlike other surrogate scenarios, you should think of any interview with the parent as an interview with the patient. When talking to parents of sick children, you always should be mindful of the emotional burdens and do not introduce information until you have established what the parent already knows. When you introduce information, speak with clarity to reduce the level of anxiety felt by the parents. Parents want to know the truth, so speak honestly, and give them the time they need to talk about their concerns. When faced with a chronic/permanent condition, most parents want to know:

- What treatment can achieve for their child in terms of relief of symptoms and prolongation of life
- How to shorten the course of the disease
- When and if they can expect progress during treatment
- What to expect by way of improvement, side effects
- Chances of complete cure
- Standard and alternative treatment options

Use empathic responses and enlist supportive services for the parent, especially in the event of bereavement. To support their role as surrogate and overcome communication challenges, you must be able to:

- Understand their concerns, problems, and beliefs
- Explain the child's illness and its treatment
- Convince parents to follow a treatment plan
- Establish a relationship with the parents and child, based on mutual respect and trust
- Use "soft skills" to put all types of parents at ease, generate confidence, and demonstrate that you are comfortable holding conversations about non-medical subjects with parents

# Talking to Children with a Sick Parent

Talking with children about their sick parents can be tricky, so it is important to follow several principals of communication with children. When you have to discuss the parent's condition, try to have the parent or caregiver present. When you initiate a discussion with a child, communicate at the level of the child's understanding. Development, not age, plays a critical role in a child's understanding of life and death. Since chronological age is an unreliable guidepost for discerning their level of understanding, do not assume anything. Instead, you should start with simple vocabulary and work your way up to more complex language if the child demonstrates an ability to comprehend complex communication. Children may ask you to repeat the message several times in order to be sure that you mean what you are saying. If they ask you to repeat something, demonstrate patience and repeat it. Very young children tend to believe in magical thinking. In other words, when a parent becomes ill, they think they may have thought or done something to cause the problem. If you detect evidence of magical thinking while talking to the child, explain that they did not do anything to cause the problem. Advising the parents to recap events from the past week is the best way to initiate a talk with children about the initial diagnosis. In the weeks following, children may react with temporary fluctuations in their behavior and mood, and especially as their parent's medical status changes. If the parent undergoes a change in treatment, explain to the child that the medicine is not working, and that you have suggested a new medicine that you hope will work better. If the child asks what will happen if the new medicine does not work, express hopefulness while acknowledging the uncertainty.

If the parent has a terminal illness, you need to prepare the child for the parent's imminent death. Again, you have to determine their understanding about death in order to formulate an approach to saying good-bye. For toddlers and preschoolers, saying goodbye might mean kissing the parent goodnight on the cheek without awareness that it is the last time. For a 10-year-old, saying goodbye might mean telling the child how much the parent loves the child. For adolescents, it might mean forgiving the child for any difficulties that existed in the relationship. In order to promote a sense of security, ask the caregiver to put the child on a regular routine so the child has a sense of normalcy. Keeping the child busy also prevents the child from thinking about the parent's sickness. When and if the parent dies, substitute terms like "death" with euphemisms like "passing on" or "went to heaven." However, be aware that spiritual descriptions may confuse children, so it is better to stick with corporeal euphemisms that children can understand. In addition to being given a clear but euphemistic description of death, children need reassurance that adults are available to love and care for them, that life will go on, and that they will not always feel sad.

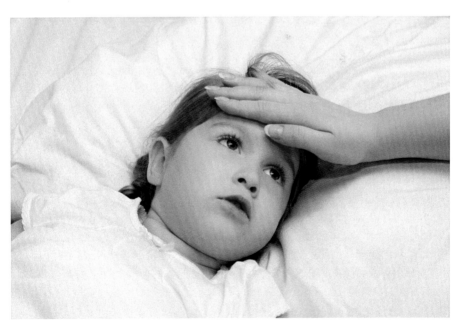

## CASE STUDY

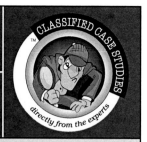

Name: Amy
Title: Children's Hospice
Program Counselor

"As the children's counselor for a hospice program, people frequently ask me to inform their children about their mother or father's terminal prognosis because people often find themselves uncertain about how to tell their children. On one occasion, a man enrolled in a hospice care program was dying and his wife asked me to help give her children the bad news. The first step was to offer empathy and support to the woman as a grieving wife before offering support in her role as mother. In formulating a plan to tell the children, I collected information on them: who they were, what they had been told, what they had observed and understood of their father's decline, as well as any religious or spiritual beliefs they had about life, death, and life after death. After obtaining this information, I initiated a discussion with the mother about her preferences. She feared being too emotional, and she requested that I tell the children of their father's coming death. I agreed, and we scheduled a home visit.

"When I arrived at the home, the patient was very weak. I explained to him the reason for my visit, and he expressed his support. Afterward, the patient's wife and I went into another room where she introduced her children. I spent time establishing rapport by showing interest in them and asking personal questions, such as their age, what school they attended, their favorite hobbies, and so forth. At this time, I began to explore their understanding of their father's illness, what they knew about it, what it has been like for them and their family during the course of his illness, and what they observed about their father's present condition. To broach this, I would ask them a question like, 'Do you think he is getting better or worse?' The children said they believed their father was getting worse, and this gave us an opportunity to talk about the reality of their father's condition (i.e. why he slept more, stayed in the bed all the time, ate less, talked less, etc.). Based on these questions, I was able to confirm what they already believed and let them know it was possible that their father could die soon. We talked about how hard their father had been fighting to get better and how hard the family was trying to help him get better. We discussed that it was not anyone's fault; their father's health was simply declining.

"Their mother listened and comforted the children as I spoke. She asked them if they understood what I told them. One of the children protested a little, saying that their father had gotten worse before, so why would he not get better again? I used an empathic response by acknowledging how difficult it is to think about their father not getting better this time. We reviewed the process of how their father's illness had progressed over the past year, and the child was able to see how much weaker and sicker the father had become this time.

"The children expressed their intention of continuing to help care for their father and the mother, and I agreed that was what they should do. We talked about different emotional responses and the importance of their expressing themselves in healthy ways by talking with trusted adults, drawing pictures, writing in a journal, allowing themselves to cry, and not being afraid to ask questions. When the children had no further questions, they went off to another room and played. I then spent the remainder of the time with their mother, talking about grief and how children at that age process information and how they will express themselves in the future. We discussed ways to continue providing support to them, emphasizing the importance of assuring her children that she would be OK, and the family would be OK as they go through this together. We ended the discussion with a conversation about teaching her children to understand the normality of feeling sadness, anger, worry, or fear from these circumstances. I made additional visits to monitor their coping status and support needs. I also was present at the time of their father's death, and provided them with one year of bereavement support after his passing."

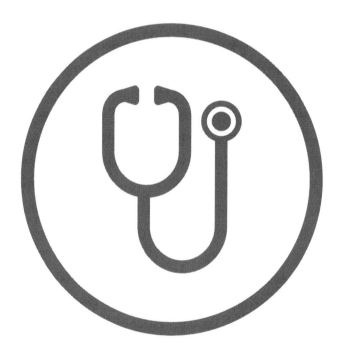

# Chapter 8

# Ethical Issues of Communication in Palliative Care

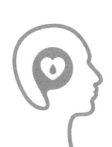

edical ethics is a system of moral principles that apply values and judgments to the practice of medicine. The first code of medical ethics called *Formula Comitis Archiatrorum,* was published in the 5th century under the Germanic rule of Theodoric the Great. Following the decline of Europe, Muslim societies furthered the foundations of ethical writ during the medieval period. The principles of medical ethics continued to grow as the western world emerged from the Dark Ages. By 1815, the British Parliament passed the Apothecaries Act, which served as the beginning of ethical regulation in modern medicine. Today, the principals of biomedical ethics exist as guidelines to help health care practitioners resolve the most common moral dilemmas presented in their relational and medical encounters with patients. Ethical and moral dilemmas may take the form of therapeutic or preventative health care decisions. Health care practitioners who fail to respect their patients' legal entitlements can face serious consequences, including fines, jail time, and the loss of their professional licenses. In their book, *Principals of Biomedical Ethics*, James Childress and Tom Beauchamp outline the four main ethical concerns of today, which include:

- Ethical concern for autonomy
- Ethical concern for beneficence
- Ethical concern for non-maleficence
- Ethical concern for justice

These four concerns require both contemplation and conversation in order to weigh the needs and desires of the patient against the moral dilemmas that those needs and desires may create. Thus, you must ask yourself, "What am I supposed to determine in the case of each ethical concern and what value does this protect?" Autonomy is a form of personal liberty. To protect autonomy, we are required to determine the wishes of the patient. Since many diseases facilitate loss of autonomy, a person's capacity to make decisions may determine their right to autonomy.

Beneficence and non-maleficence are slightly different principles that frequently go hand-in-hand. Beneficence is moral obligation to act for the benefit of others by preventing or removing possible harms. Put another way, beneficence means that unless there is a sufficient reason to the contrary, you have an obligation to make decisions that are likely to do more good than harm. Some ethics scholars such as Edmund Pellegrino argue that beneficence is the only relevant principle of medical ethics because healing should be the sole purpose of medicine. Some of these scholars argue that peripheral health-related industries in cosmetic surgery, contraception, and euthanasia do not fall under the aegis of ethical concern, providing evidence that the philosophy of medical ethics is open to some degree of interpretation.

Non-maleficence is the principle of avoiding harm. Since the legal definition of non-maleficence differs depending on the cultural, religious, political, legal, or social beliefs of the culture where you practice medicine, you should not consider non-maleficence a matter of interpretation. Any violation of non-maleficence may subject you to medical malpractice litigation. Therefore, in order to protect the principles of beneficence and non-maleficence, we must determine the patient's views of what values need to be protected, what harms need to be avoided, and what regulations, if any, exist that prevent you from protecting these values.

According to Beauchamp and Childress, when there is a conflict between the principles of beneficence and non-maleficence, the principle of non-maleficence trumps the principle of beneficence. For example, let us suppose you have an immediate need for an organ donor for a patient on dialysis, and you have a patient on life support with two working kidneys, non-maleficence dictates that you should not harvest the kidneys of the patient on life support to save the life of the patient on dialysis. If you offer treatment, as another example, and your patient rejects the treatment, the patient's informed decision to reject treatment overrides your recommendation. If you cannot tell what benefits or harms the patient, some ethicists argue that you should distinguish medical benefits from quality-of-life benefits. Others argue that the two are interrelated. Either way, it is worth noting that code 2.17 of the American Medical Association recognizes the legitimacy of quality-of-life considerations when making treatment decisions. To determine what constitutes a "quality-of-life as a medical benefit" consideration, give the most weight to what the patient sees as the most beneficial effect of treatment.

The principle of justice concerns the larger ethical needs of the community. For example, justice may concern the distribution of scarce health resources, and the decision of who gets what treatment. According to Beauchamp and Childress, the principle of justice requires you to treat the same types of medical cases equally, with the same treatment. Medical need should be determined in terms of the benefit to the patient, the urgency of need, the change in quality of life, and the duration of benefit. Ethically, you should not weigh for consideration any non-medical aspects such as the ability to pay for care, social class, treatment obstacles, or the patient's contribution to their illness. However, given the difficulty of being able to account for fair distribution of equal health care, consider calling for an open discussion of rationing policies to ensure that rationing limits have at least gone through a process of reaching a general consensus. Regardless of any limitations, it is important to follow due process in order to determine and accept the limits of health care on an individual case basis. The need for ethical conversations about justice between doctors and patients may be necessary when medical limitations appear. In his book, *The Foundations of Bioethics*, Tristam Englehardt argues that patients and health care practitioners come to a clinical relationship as moral strangers who need to negotiate moral arrangements, and that health care practitioners must become the moral negotiators using the four ethical concerns to govern their approach. If you work in an emergency room or military hospital, resource allocation should adhere to the medical triage model of ethics to bring about the greatest good in a situation of scarcity. Therefore, you should base resource allocation according to medical need and priority. On an individual level, code 2.03 of the American Medical Association states that you should not ration at the bedside because it inevitably violates the principle of justice and the demand for due process in establishing rationing policies.

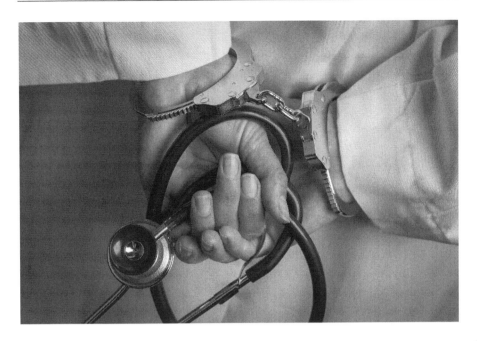

In some cases, you may find that moral reasoning cannot guide ethical decisions. The alternative approach to moral reasoning is "casuistry," which asserts that moral knowledge develops incrementally through analysis of specific cases. Casuistry stands as a judgment model where the task is simply to find the right answer to any given moral problem, free of established guidelines. Because some problems may not clearly fall under the strictures of law, the solution to the problem may require a kind of moral relativism. Richard Miller's *Casuistry and Modern Ethics* advises that any casuist approach to unique ethical dilemmas should attempt to draw on existing paradigms, relevant presumptions, extenuating circumstances, and the moral options of prior experts in order to reach a verdict on ethical responsibility. When ethical principles fall into conflict, consider the approach of virtue ethics. Virtue ethics can provide a flexible approach to a solution when none other appears viable. This principle considers the virtues of character as a means of determining or evaluating the solution to a dilemma. For example, some health practitioners might consider lying to be unethical, whereas a virtue ethicist might consider what lying says about their own character and moral behavior. If any guidelines exist for the virtue ethicist, they are not established strictures of law but rather virtuous characteristics such as compassion, practical wisdom, sincerity, trustworthiness, honesty, conscientiousness, and competence.

# The Doctrine of Informed Consent

The doctrine of informed consent states that you must fully inform patients about their health status if they are mentally competent enough to understand it. According to the American Association of Neurological Surgeons, "The legal doctrine is primarily concerned with liabilities associated with breach. Breach of the doctrine of informed consent may be actionable… Informed consent claims are often coupled with a claim for medical malpractice and typically arise when a patient experiences an adverse outcome from a treatment or surgery. The standard allegation in a claim for lack of informed consent is that the doctor never informed the patient, or inadequately informed the patient, about the possibility of the adverse outcome. The majority of informed consent claims turn on the element of causation. To prove causation and ultimately succeed on such a claim, the patient must demonstrate that [the doctor did not disclose the possibility of an adverse outcome, and the patient would not have chosen to proceed with the treatment or surgery if the doctor had done so.]" The doctrine derives from the principles of autonomy, beneficence, non-maleficence, and justice. Informed consent can occur in either written or oral form, and contains five elements, which include:

- Discussion about the reason for making a medical decision
- Communication of its potential benefits
- Understanding of the risks
- Discussion about alternatives
- Understanding that the decision is voluntary

# The Goals of Informed Consent

With respect to informed consent, Beauchamp and Childress recommend three possible standards of approach: the reasonable patient standard, the reasonable physician standard, and the subjective standard. The reasonable patient standard asks what kind of information the average patient must ethically receive in order to make an informed decision about their health. The reasonable physician standard asks what the average physician believes is the ethical decision to make about informed consent. The subjective standard, similar to casuistry, examines the uniqueness of each medical case and asks what *specific* information the physician is ethically required to give the patient in order to make an informed decision. However, you should be aware that the subjective standard invalidates any blanket waivers signed by the patient, which allows the health care provider to release medical information to government agencies, insurance companies, employers, and others.

Determining the best ethical approach to informed consent requires reexamination of the ethical concerns (autonomy, beneficence, nonmaleficence, and justice). To determine a patient's level of autonomy, you must find the moral basis behind the patient's right to self-rule. Since the principle of autonomy directly translates into the principle of informed consent, you must follow the doctrine of informed consent to affirm autonomy. In order to affirm the patient's autonomy, first examine the requirements of informed consent. To meet the requirements of informed consent, the patient or surrogate must:

- Be capable of understanding consequences and capable of making a free choice
- Be free from coercion or undue influence
- Demonstrate mental competence to make medical decisions that require: knowing that he or she is authorizing medical

treatment, understanding of the treatment's range of effects, understanding of alternative options in terms of health, life, lifestyle, religious beliefs, values, family, friends, and all other factors bearing on treatment decisions

To fulfill the obligation of informed consent, the physician must:

- Provide and make understandable necessary information for making a free, intelligent treatment decision
- Facilitate a reflective conversation with the patient to check for understanding
- Recommend what the physician believes is the optimal option without pressuring the patient into making this decision
- Provide known alternatives
- Include the hospital's success and failure rates with the proposed treatment
- Understand that legal informed consent (e.g. asking the patient to sign a waiver) differs from the moral standards of informed consent

After you honor your obligation to informed consent, make every effort to discuss and document any relevant aspects of the four ethical concerns in the patient's medical records, including their preferences.

However, when it comes to assessing incompetence, there is no established protocol except through gradual assessments of the patient via medical interviews. Beauchamp and Childress suggest looking for several qualifiers, which include the inability to express preferences, the inability to understand one's situation and its consequences, the inability to understand relevant information, the inability to provide rational answers to questions, and the inability to make reasonable decisions. However, one caveat exists when making competency assessments.

For example, if the patient has values that differ from the health care provider's values, this alone does not prove incompetence. If we assert through the moral reasoning of casuistry that moral knowledge develops incrementally through analysis of specific cases, there may be some cases where the standards for competence may be set higher if the consequences are more substantial.

If you determine the patient or surrogate decision-maker to be incompetent, consult any documented known prior preferences (such as a living will) to see if any decision-making instructions were built into the document. If no will exists, consult the next available surrogate decision maker using the previously mentioned Family Health Care Decisions Act available in Appendix J. According to Beauchamp, any estimates made by the next available surrogate decision maker "requires substantial information about the patient's views and wishes and must not simply reflect the preferences or interests of the physician or surrogate… If no sufficient basis to make a substituted judgment exists, the physician or surrogate must decide based on his or her judgment about what would be in the best interest of the patient. Estimates of best interest are based on what a rational, normal person would prefer, not just on what the physician or surrogate prefers."

If disagreement exists between acting parties, call those in dissent to exchange information and views. If the decision involves an ethical dilemma, ask the hospital chaplain, family priest, minister, or rabbi to attend the meeting as a facilitator for reaching agreement. If the meeting does not result in consensus, consult your hospital's institutional ethics committee. If a surrogate or physician is acting against the expressed preferences of the patient and the institutional ethics committee fails to bring a resolution of the disagreement, you may consult the courts to order treatment or appoint a conservator.

While this may seem like a lot of red tape, it is important to remember that you are protecting yourself from legal consequences in addition to doing what is in the best interest of the patient. With respect to the pursuit of informed consent, certain exceptions exist, and you may encounter them on an individual basis. If a procedure is non-invasive or risky by legal consideration, you do not need to fulfill any obligation to informed consent. If by way of evidence you have reason to believe that information will adversely affect the patient's condition or health, you may be entitled to withhold that information. If the patient is not mentally competent during an emergency medical situation in which the patient's life is in danger and no prior preferences are available, the law waives you from the obligation to seek informed consent. If the patient demands immediate treatment and you have reason to believe it may create an irreversible consequence, you may be justified in postponing treatment on the ethical concern of beneficence. Suggested further readings on the doctrine of informed consent include *A History and Theory of Informed Consent* by Tom Beauchamp and Ruth Faden and *Informed Consent: Legal Theory and Clinical Practice* by Jessica Berg *(et al)*.

# Ethical Issues in the Use of Decision Aids

The use of decision aids in steering patients toward their choices raises ethical questions, as some researchers believe they have the propensity to distort decisions if patients inappropriately weigh certain aspects of information instead of considering all aspects of information relevant to their individual case. Research of patients who use decision aids seems to suggest that patients feel more satisfied with decisions made intuitively rather than analytically. In a 2007 report by Wendy L. Nelson (*et al.*) titled *Rethinking the Objectives of Decision Aids: A Call for Conceptual Clarity*, studies found that "when many facets of a decision problem need to be considered and compared, conscious thought is less efficient and more likely to [create too much emphasis on one particular attribute] than unconscious thought. Unconscious thought, on the other hand, is more adept at forming global impressions, which is useful when multiple attributes need consideration."

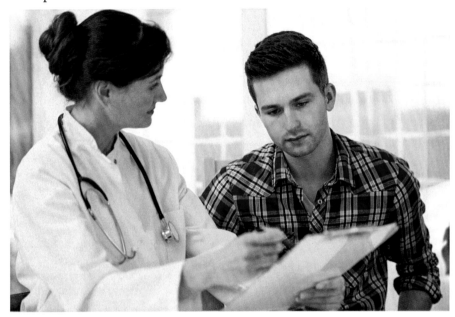

Decision aids, therefore, may create unintended bias due to over-scrutinization. In order to fulfill your ethical obligations to informed consent, you must not use decision aids as a means of backing your medical opinions, but rather, as a means of providing the patient with as much information as possible to reach informed consent. Decision aids take two approaches to elicit values and determine the patient's preferences and strength of options. The first approach involves clinical scenarios describing the options and outcomes of health. The second entails the use of value clarification exercises, which the patient interacts with after considering all the relevant information about each option. These exercises include utility assessment, probability tradeoff tasks, social matching, weight scale exercises, relevance charts, and analytic hierarchy process methods.

As a physician, you must be careful how you use these aids. Using decision aids as a means of steering the patient toward one decision or another is coercion. Coercion happens when the doctor does not allow the patient to come to their own decision, but rather, uses various methods to bring about a desired choice. For example, if you offer a decision aid, but do not state your views on clinical trial participation, patients may feel pressured to participate. You can remedy leaving the patient with ambiguous opinions that pressure them into coercion by simply changing the language of your communication. For example, saying "you are eligible for this trial" implies that the patient is lucky and should seize the opportunity. However, saying "This trial may be suitable for you" implies that the trial is a possible option without implying that the patient should try to meet the criteria for the trial. Keep in mind that a fine line exists between persuasion and coercion. When patients are already leaning toward a decision, having done so on their own accord, using a decision aid to persuade them in the direction they are leaning is not considered coercion. Informed consent of clinical trials means that the patient must understand the diagnosis, the relationship between the illness and their future health, and the benefits of standard therapy options. A decision aid also may fail to point out the differences between how the patient would receive therapy in clinical vs. standard treatments.

Decision aids can create coercion, especially if the patient has no particular values in mind for his or her medical treatment. If the patient has to make a decision in haste, the physician may be tempted to coerce the patient into making a decision he or she is not ready to make. In such cases, a decision aid is not likely to help patients choose in a way that is consistent with their personal values. According to Nelson, "a large and growing body of research suggests that factors such as low numeracy, biases in information presentation (e.g., framing effects and order effects), and heuristic reasoning influence information processing and judgment…Clarifying personal values is a central task in decision-making under uncertainty." Studies cited by Nelson indicate that it is not clear that decision aids — as they currently exist — can or should be used to perform this task. Therefore, the most effective and ethical use of decision aids would be to involve these aids as a purely supplementary form of information, free of coercion.

# Ethical Issues in Shared Decision-Making

While shared decision-making is currently the most accepted type of doctor-patient relationship, the responsibilities that come with it can compromise your ethical boundaries if you are not careful. Since shared decision-making means that both the patient and physician offer their input into the decision-making process, there are times when both parties have to reach a compromise in their values. However, what do you do when a patient asks you to compromise your *ethical* values? For instance, if a patient asked you for a prescription that you know they will use to hasten his or her death, your ethical values face compromise. Whenever you encounter a situation whereby the patient's values are forcing you to compromise your ethical values as a health care practitioner, the best course of action is to:

1. Acknowledge the patient's terrible situation
2. Discuss the legitimacy of the request
3. Engage the patient in a conversation about your own emotional response to such a request

The third step in this process is important because when patients make requests that compromise ethical responsibilities, they have done so without considering the consequences it may have to others. Using the previous example, if a patient requested a lethal prescription to end their suffering, you would use the third step in this process to talk about how you would not be able to live with yourself if you allowed the request. When patients realize their actions have an effect on others, they begin to understand the conflict between the physician's responsibility to the patient and to the concept of right and wrong. Giving the patient a clear understanding of your ethical responsibilities will more often than not allow the doctor-patient relationship to continue. At the very least, the patient will emerge from this conversation feeling that you listened to their fears and concerns.

# Mental Capacity Act of 1983

There are some medical cases where it is obvious that the patient is not mentally capable of understanding medical information or making informed choices. For example, if a patient has a mental illness or medication that limits his or her capacity to act of sound mind, you have to be able to judge the limits of their mental capacity in order to ascertain the validity of the patient's decisions. Disclosing medical information to a patient in a delirious state puts the doctor in the difficult position of trying to figure out if the patient's consent is truly informed. In 1983, the United Kingdom introduced the Mental Capacity Act, which covers the reception, care, and treatment of mentally disordered persons. Under the Mental Capacity Act — most recently amended in 2007 — people diagnosed with a mental disorder can be detained in hospital or police custody and have their disorder assessed or treated against their wishes. Mental capacity under this law designates the term "capacity" as subject to fluctuation, therefore you must continually test the patient's ability to understand the choices made on his or her behalf. If you determine the patient to be permanently impaired, you must communicate with the patient in simple language and create a stress-free environment. If mental capacity shows no signs of improvement, you are required to consult with either someone with the power of attorney, family members, and/ or surrogate decision makers to inform them of the patient's status. If you find such an individual assigned to the charge of caregiver or surrogate decision maker, you must register them formally in that role and make clear to them that they cannot override any advanced directive consented to by the patient in a mentally capable state. While physicians in the United States and other western countries use the doctrine of informed consent to guide such actions, the United Kingdom's Mental Capacity Act provides a responsible reference point for fulfilling professional obligation and protecting the patient's rights. Five statutory principals underpin the legislation of the Mental Capacity Act:

1. You must assume someone has mental capacity before you establish otherwise.
2. You must not treat the patient as unable to make a decision unless you have taken all measures to determine them incapable of making decisions.
3. You must not confuse poor decisions with the inability to make decisions.
4. You must act on behalf of the patient's best interests.
5. You must be as unrestrictive to the patient's rights as possible when acting on behalf of the patient's best interests.

# Ethical Concerns about Enrollment in Clinical Trials

To elaborate further on the concept of coercion, physicians are ethically responsible to offer their treatment preference when an informed person has no enrollment preference between two recommended treatment options. The condition by which patients express no preference between treatments is individual equipoise. Ethical law does not consider persuasion to be an act of coercion in cases where the patient demonstrates individual equipoise. However, if the patient demonstrates individual equipoise, and the physician considers one treatment more effective over another, the principal of beneficence applies and the doctor is ethically required to provide his or her recommendation. Since clinical trials are more likely to yield uncertainties, it is ethically acceptable for the physician to defer control of the treatment decision to a randomization process. In other words, if the patient has no treatment preference between two clinical trials, and the physician has no empirical evidence to recommend one trial over another, the physician may let the patient randomly choose the treatment following fulfillment of informed consent.

Before you allow your ambivalent patients to choose their enrollment program, you should first know if the larger medical community practices individual or collective equipoise. Collective equipoise means that a best practice standard among doctors supersedes the notion of individual equipoise. Collective equipoise gives a group of doctors the right to override individual equipoise, even if the individual doctor prefers one treatment to another for the patient. The medical community justifies this override on the premise that the certainties regarding clinical trials may change at any time and yield newly discovered dangers from the clinical trial research. If your patients experience negative side effects in a clinical trial, you should report this newly discovered danger to the medical community immediately so they may enforce collective equipoise on that clinical trial.

As of this writing, the question of collective equipoise in randomized trials remains a controversy. In their research report titled, *Does Clinical Equipoise Apply to Cluster Randomized Trials in Health Research?* by Ariella Binik (*et al*), it was found that "randomized trial interventions often target health care providers rather than patients and may have only an indirect impact on patient care." To assuage the problem of collective equipoise, researchers suggest that control group subjects undergo a minimal amount of experimental intervention. In addition, implementation of early stopping rules in randomized trials can help to resolve ethical concerns about data favoring the experimental treatment generated during a trial. According to Binik, "The trust relationship between state and research subjects has two central advantages. First, recognition of this trust relationship provides a foundation for clinical equipoise, which does not depend on a pre-existing relationship between a physician-researcher and a patient-subject. As a result, this trust relationship [applies] clinical equipoise to the resolution of ethical tension in randomized trials. Second, it helps to specify the role and obligations of research ethics committees in the ethical analysis of risk in CRT as well as in all RCTs."

Simply put, collective equipoise raises ethical questions due to the distinctions made between research and therapy. Clinical research involves conflict between developing scientific knowledge and protecting research participants from harm. The reason for this conflict resides in the fact that clinical research is not a therapeutic activity devoted to the personal care of patients. Since the research investigators' goals are not primarily concerned with therapy, the inherent potential of exploiting test subjects in clinical trials always exists. Therefore, if your patient chooses to enroll in a clinical trial, your job as an arbiter of informed consent is to make clear the distinction between the goals of the clinical trial's investigators and the goal of the patient to gain a therapeutic benefit. When you research the efficacy of a clinical trial, consider an ethical evaluation system as part of your evaluation. A 2003 Hastings Center report by Franklin Miller and Howard Brody devised an ethical framework of requirements for all clinical research, which include ethical evaluation of:

- The trial's scientific or social value (the potential for widespread use)
- The trial's scientific validity (building on foundations of legitimate science)

- The researchers' methods of fair subject selection (no evidence that suggests vulnerable patients were inappropriately recruited)
- The trial's favorable risk-benefit ratio (risks to participants not excessive and are justified by the knowledge to be gained from the research)
- Independent reviews of the trial (approval from an ethics review board and proof that enrolled subjects gave informed consent)
- Informed consent (documented proof)
- Enrolled research participants' review of the trials (permission to speak with enrolled subjects)

# Recruitment Barriers in Clinical Trials

Gaining informed consent to clinical trials can present a challenge due to the conflicting goals of the researchers and your goal of doing what is right for the patient's health. Being mindful of the two diverging goals is important because you risk damaging your relationship with the patient if the clinical trial adversely affects the patient's health. Statistically, the number of eligible patients who decline a clinical trial ranges between 23 to 50 percent, according to a 1984 study by J.F. Martin in the *American Journal of Clinical Oncology*. Reasons that patients cite include their perceptions of experimentation, loss of control, and uncertainty of outcome. Physicians who do not enroll their patients in clinical trials cite rigid protocols, inconveniences to the patient, and the extra work involved.

# Gaining Informed Consent to Clinical Trials

If you choose to discuss enrollment into clinical trials with your patient, you must focus on what and how you tell your patients about the trials. You can achieve both by providing all the information on the consent document, such as the legal aspects of the study protocol and the potential adverse effects, including side effects. In his 2004 medical journal, *Developing Ethical Strategies to Assist Oncologists in Seeking Informed Consent to Cancer Clinical Trials*, Richard Brown found that studies of patients confronted with the option of clinical trials identified participation in treatment decision-making as an essential component to seeking informed consent to the clinical trial. To facilitate a discussion of clinical trials, use the shared decision-making model and SEGUE framework. Brown suggests 14 strategies for encouraging collaborative decision-making, which include:

- Introducing the joint decision-making process
- Using language that reflects patient autonomy
- Checking preferred decision-making style (involved or not)
- Checking information preferences of patient
- Inviting questions and comments
- Checking medical knowledge of patient
- Checking patient understanding
- Explicitly offering choice of treatment
- Acknowledging uncertainty of treatment benefits
- Declaring professional recommendation
- Providing opportunity for amplification of patient voice
- Providing time and opportunity to discuss patient concerns in detail
- Offering decision delay
- Offering ongoing decision support/answers to future questions

Using the prescribed strategies, Brown recommends a ten-step protocol. Assuming that you already have used your "bearings" to orient the patient into an understanding of the illness, the first step toward gaining consent to a clinical trial involves the "pathway" phase. The pathway phase involves the initial discussion of standard treatments. Discussion of standard treatment must always precede any discussion of clinical trials. Once you have discussed the standard treatment, the next phase is "amplification." Amplification involves giving the patient a chance to react to the standard treatment options. The third phase is "declaration." In the declaration phase, the doctor clarifies which standard treatment he or she feels is the best among the ones presented. This gives way to the fourth phase, "enunciation." Enunciation is the point at which the patient formally articulates his or her preference among the standard treatments.

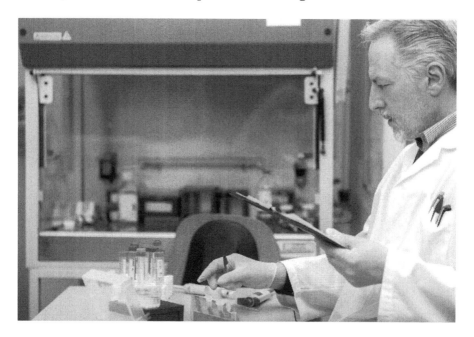

Using the SEGUE framework, you would then transition toward a discussion of clinical trials, following the same format of the previous five steps. In pathway 2, you would present the clinical trial as another treatment option and draw comparisons between the clinical trial and the preferred standard treatment option. Framing discussion in pathway 2 involves a general explanation of clinical trials, how they work, their rationale, and an explanation of the current clinical trial. If you incorporate how the trial relates to the four ethical principles outlined in this chapter (autonomy, beneficence, non-maleficence, and justice), you will be that much closer to gaining the patient's confidence and consent to the trial. Once you provide your explanations, amplification 2 provides an opportunity for the patient to express their opinion and concerns about the information. After the patient offers their reaction, use declaration 2 to emphasize the fact that the patient's decision will not influence your clinical relationship. Enunciation 2 gives the patient the opportunity to make a formal decision between the preferred standard treatment and the clinical trial option. The final step is enactment, whereby the doctor begins to execute the shared decision and describes the next steps in the treatment process. Figure 12 provides a visual example of the ten-step process, using the SEGUE framework to transition from the discussion of standard treatment to clinical trials.

### *Figure 12. Discussing Clinical Trial Enrollment*

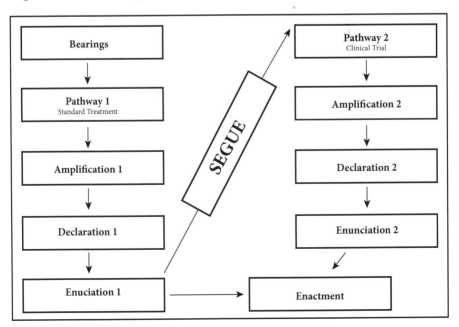

# Communication Risks of CAM Treatment

Before your patient decides to choose their preferred treatment in the second enunciation of your discussion, you can always introduce a third option: complementary and alternative medicine, otherwise known as CAM. Complementary and alternative medicine is the term for medical products and practices that are not part of standard care. It is important that you explain the difference between complementary and alternative medicine. Alternative medicine takes the place of standard medical care and is not necessarily a clinical trial. An example of alternative medicine is treating heart disease with chelation therapy (which seeks to remove excess metals from the blood) instead of using a standard approach. Complementary medicine, on the other hand, is any medicine that you combine with standard medical care. Medicine considered complementary also must have a proven record of safety and effectiveness. An example of complementary medicine is the use of acupuncture to help with side effects of cancer treatment. Even if you do not believe CAM treatments to be effective, it may serve the principal of beneficence and non-maleficence if the patient believes the treatment will help. In any clinical encounter with serious illness, it is important to sometimes take a contextual approach and understand that factors unique to the patient's life may be at work in their decisions. For example, the patient may have concerns about the cost of care, and may want to use a less costly alternative medicine, or they may believe a complementary medicine will have double the treatment effect. To communicate the risks of treatment, the *Handbook of Communication in Oncology and Palliative Care* recommends the following steps:

- Elicit the patient's understanding of their illness and clarify their information preferences

- Respect cultural or social beliefs
- Ask the patient if he or she is considering any CAM medicines to treat side effects
- Ask the patient about the CAM (how often it's supposed to be used, what they hope to achieve, if there is any research proving its effectiveness)
- Provide some evidence-based knowledge of the CAM
- Help the patient respond to advice about CAM from family and friends
- Respond to the patient's emotional state
- Discuss relevant concerns about CAM such as financial cost, psychological risks, and any unknown effects
- Establish a trial period to evaluate its benefit and efficacy
- Consider making a referral to a CAM practitioner
- Encourage CAM use if studies indicate low risk and discourage if studies indicate evidence that it is unsafe while balancing advice with acknowledgment of patient's right to autonomy
- Summarize the main points of your discussion about CAM
- Document the discussion
- Follow up on your discussion about CAM in the next consultation

# Discussing Fertility Risk Issues

Serious illness sometimes requires conversations about fertility risks from aggressive treatments such as chemotherapy and radiation. A 2004 study published by B.J. Zebrak in *Psycho-Oncology* found that 60 percent of young adult survivors of childhood cancer reported uncertainty about their fertility status because only half the health care providers discussed potential reproductive problems associated with aggressive treatments.

To avoid patient dissatisfaction later, discussion of any potential fertility risk from therapies should come before your patient reaches the enunciation stage. You can accomplish this by providing clear, factual information about any known risks in both in written and verbal form. You also should include significant others who would be affected by reproduction problems and provide cryopreservation directions with referrals to sperm banks. Above all, keep the fertility discussion ongoing throughout the course of treatment.

## CASE STUDY

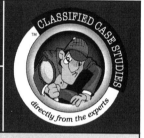

Name: Amy Brodkey, M.D.
Title: Addiction Psychiatrist
State: Pennsylvania

**Excerpt Taken From:** A Questions of Ethics: An Expert Interview with Amy Brodkey, MD, **www.medscape.com/viewarticle/713480**

Medicine is fraught with questions relating to the ethics of relationships between physicians and industry. A physician's primary fiduciary duty is to patients and their well-being. A competing interest can lie in accepting gifts, payment above the normal salary, or doing anything else for self-gain that conflicts with your duty to patients, students, or the public health. The effects of conflicts of interest are often subtle, and a doctor may not even realize that it is affecting how he or she practices. Industry's aim is to make money for their stockholders. Relationships with industry can conflict with a doctor's duty. Numerous studies show that industry influence on physicians frequently leads to harm — not only to patients, but also to trainees, the public, and the profession.

Many physicians do not meet with pharmaceutical representatives anymore because they are marketers, not educators. The best way to reduce conflicts of interest is to distance oneself as much as possible. There is also the opinion that if someone speaks for several drug companies, you can trust them more. The reality is that sponsors vet content beforehand. The question is absurd. Why should you get your information from sources that you know are biased? For those of us who work in impoverished areas and take uninsured patients, drug samples are tempting, but there are harms to using them. Drug companies do not sample generic or older products; they sample the newest and most expensive medications. Studies show that samples are rarely the doctor's first choice. If you give those out, patients will probably stay on the same medication once they become insured, running up health care costs.

We also know very little about the long-term safety of new drugs. Studies show that a large portion of samples actually are used by health care workers and their families, and do not reach patients...Disclosure is important, but we know very little about its effects. Often, disclosure is ignored and people do not know what to disclose. Psychology research shows that biased advice is frequently unintended and unconsciously motivated. Some people who disclose may exaggerate claims, or they may feel less responsible for accuracy because they disclosed information. Some evidence suggests that people often underestimate how severely conflict of interest affects them.

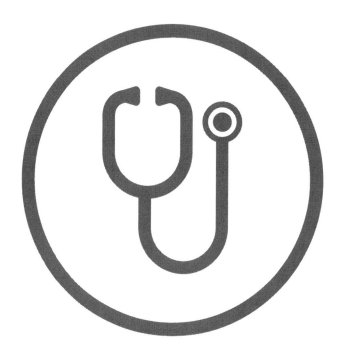

# Chapter 9

# Transitioning Patients to Palliative Care

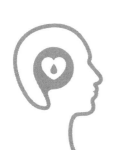

When the treatment of disease requires you to consider shifting the patient from curative care to palliative care, your challenge is breaking the news that curative care is not working, helping the patient to accept this fact, and recommending a shift to palliative care. The transition from curative care to palliative care is about changing the overall goals of the patient's health care. In other words, if the overall goal of curative care is to cure the patient of the disease, then the overall goal of palliative care is to provide relief from the symptoms of an incurable disease and improve the quality of life for the patient and the family. This means recognizing that you have exhausted all treatment options, and that management of the disease requires a radical change in the patient's goals and expectations. If you tell your patient that curative treatments have failed, the patient may revert into highly-charged emotional states along the extended grief cycle. Your job is to alleviate the patient's uncertainty using the principles outlined in this book and explain how palliative care works.

*Figure 13. Palliative Care Transitions*

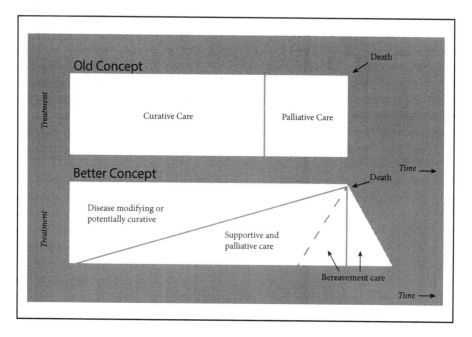

Most conversations about transitioning to palliative care are difficult because no clear boundaries exist between curative and palliative care, and many physicians and nurses often lack the knowledge of what this specialized service actually involves. The use of palliative care services vary depending on the needs of the patient and the palliative resources available. Some patients use palliative care specialists to help them manage the entire scope of care while others enlist the services of their primary care physician. The best way to brace your patients for palliative care is to have an early conversation about illness trajectories, explore the possibility of transitioning from curative to palliative if all treatment options fail, and provide an early referral to a palliative care specialist. If the patient's disease progresses unabated, you will then be able to ease the patient gradually into a transition rather than into a transition that comes as a complete surprise. Figure 13 illustrates the difference between a sharp transition (old concept), which contributes to distress, and a gradual transition (new concept), which helps to alleviate the patient's uncertainties.

# When to Introduce the Idea of Palliative Care

The process of transitioning patients to palliative care can occur in four ways: through a conversation about the need to change the goals of care, by referral to a palliative specialist, as a result of ineffective life-extending treatments, or when the patient reaches the terminal phase of their illness. Discussing palliative care requires clear and sensitive communication, therefore you must be able to identify when it is time to talk about changing the goals of care. Patients often give us verbal "triggers" that they understand that things are not improving and are ready for a discussion about it. For example, they might start making comments about how treatments do not appear to be working. Perhaps they might talk about the burden they feel responsible for causing to family members. They also might intimate thoughts of suicide or talk about having reached the limit of their ability to tolerate pain. To approximate how long a patient has left to live, monitor the illness trajectory by your own methods (or consult the palliative care indicator tool in Appendix K). As the trajectory brings the patient closer to the final declining state of the illness, try to introduce palliative care gradually before recommending it. At this point, you already should have highlighted palliative care, however brief, during the initial consultation. Failing to have an early or gradual discussion of palliative care may otherwise leave you with an ethical dilemma. For example, in Chapter 4 we discussed how some illnesses trajectories allow the patient to maintain comfort and functioning for a substantial period, followed by a short and rapid decline. Suddenly you have a difficult choice. Do you allow the patient to live without the distress of knowing that the end is near, or do you tell the patient he or she has roughly one to three months to live? Since it would be unethical to deprive the patient of autonomy and the family a chance to make near-death preparations, you have an obligation to be frank. Introducing palliative care before it is necessary to discuss prepares everyone involved for the possibility of having to shift goals and expectations, avoids the shock of sudden decline, reduces the expensive cost of futile care, and avails you of having to deal with an ethical dilemma.

# How to Discuss Changing or Stopping Treatments

In order to introduce a conversation about palliative care, you have to break the news that treatments are not working. When patients learn about disease progression, be prepared for emotional reactions. Providing empathic support is crucial because it will allow you to segue into a discussion about changing or ending treatments. If the conversation is about changing treatments, you must be clear about the goals of treatment and what specific outcomes to expect (i.e. symptom relief). If you believe that this change in treatment may not improve the chances of survival, let the patient know. Instead of dwelling on survival, emphasize the quality of life benefits that the new treatment will provide. Provide clear information about side effects, cost, and the amount of time needed to administer it so the patient can make an informed decision in relation to their own goals. Reassure the patient that full supportive care is available and explore their desired level of involvement in the decision-making process. If the conversation is about ending treatments, explain that the disease is no longer responding to the current treatment and that continuing it is likely to cause increasingly negative side effects. Explain to the patient that it is likely that he or she will have a better quality of life by ending the treatment and transitioning toward palliative goals of symptom relief.

# Strategy for Discussing Transition to Palliative Care

Once you recognize the patient's emerging clinical reality and sit them down for a discussion, do not convey the idea that you can do nothing more for the patient. Instead, begin the interview in an appropriate setting by declaring your agenda items and negotiating what to talk about regarding the patient's situation. Next, explain the progression of the disease and offer a prognosis based on what you have negotiated to disclose. Afterward, allow the patient to express their emotions and to re-explore their goals. You can achieve this by eliciting questions and checking the patient for understanding. At this point, introduce the palliative approach. For example, you might ask what the term "palliative care" means to the patient and use this to clarify any misconceptions such as explaining that palliative care is not solely for people with terminal disease. Once you have defined the basics of palliative care, discuss the role of the palliative care team and emphasize their expertise is symptom management. At this point, allow the patient an opportunity to express an emotion; this response should tell you whether the patient is ready to talk about the process of dying. If the patient is not ready, ask open questions and allow them to explore the nature of their emotions further. It is important that you acknowledge, validate, and normalize these emotions as a way of allowing them to accept the new reality. If they appear ready to talk about the process of dying, focus the discussion on what constitutes good symptom control with detailed information and begin to explore how the transition to palliative care will affect the patient and the patient's family. In order to promote understanding of this change, validate the patient's responses, address the caregiver's concerns, summarize the discussion, and express a willingness to help by offering your services to help the patient control the symptoms and help the family cope with the new agenda.

Rather than using negative connotations to describe the agenda, frame the goals of care with positive words. For example, instead of saying "Our goal is to reduce the pain you will experience as you become sicker," you might say something like, "Our goal is to optimize your comfort and ability to function as the disease progresses." In order to promote hope over grief and despair, you should likewise talk in terms of the present rather than the future. If you cannot provide palliative care, or the patient needs a palliative care specialist, tell the patient that you work closely with a palliative care team that specializes in treating the disease. Be sure to use the term "palliative care" and explicitly state whether this palliative care team will provide the bulk of support or additional support to what you will provide. While describing what palliative specialists do, pay attention to verbal or nonverbal signs of confusion and check for understanding. Before you talk about support services, make sure you know everything about the specialist's range of support services, including support to both family and children. Otherwise, the patient may doubt the recommendation and your veracity. If you initiate a patient into palliative care before discussing an end to curative care, you might explain that the palliative care team can provide support while the patient continues to receive curative treatments. Add that you will remain the primary care provider while the patient begins to receive support service from the palliative care team, and clarify which provider will handle which issue.

# Five Emphasis Points of the Palliative Care Setting

When you talk to the patient about the palliative care setting and how it works, you should form your explanation around five points of emphasis: the role of the physician, the reason for a palliative referral, the function of a multi-disciplinary team, how to cope in palliative care, and the involvement of families in a palliative setting. In intensive care units, the switch from curative to palliative care is often dramatic and easy for clinicians to identify. In primary care settings, the transition is usually less dramatic, discrete, and identifiable. Instead of trying to recognize the moment when this transition should occur, develop an awareness of key elements in a disease's progression that occur long before the necessity of palliative care service. Early recognition of these key elements warrants initial consideration for a need to change goals and prompts a gradual move toward transition.

Primary care physicians play a critical role in guiding patients through the early stages of an illness that eventually becomes terminal. How well these physicians handle the communication and decision-making early in the clinical relationship affects the transition to palliative care. According to a 2001 study by Anthony Back and J. Randall Curtis in the *Western Journal of Medicine*, "Studies suggest that major gaps exist between what patients at the end of their life want from their medical care and what they receive. Patients say they want to die at home, but 60 percent to 80 percent die in an institution." In other words, when the central focus shifts to quality of life and symptom management, attention must be shifted to patients' subjective experience. According to Back and Curtis, physicians need to broaden their field of competence to address these gaps by developing effective skills such as communication and emotional support. To facilitate consultations that support the patient's subjective experience during this process, see the eight-step protocol outlined later in this chapter.

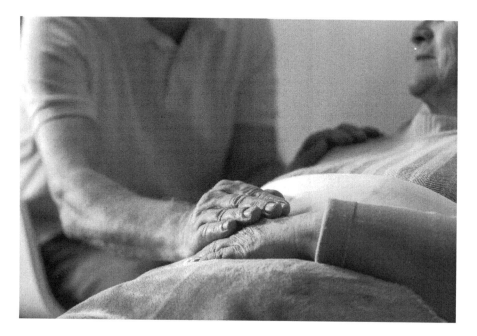

Once you have covered your role in the palliative care process, your communication necessitates a conversation on the primary reason for why you would like to make a referral to a palliative care specialist. Your explanation should cover the different reasons why physicians refer their patients to palliative care, and how hospice care relates to palliative care. A palliative care specialist will cover this kind of information in further detail, but it is important to show the patient that you are committed to their care and not simply handing them off to another doctor. In the United States, hospice is the best-known delivery model for palliative care. While hospice care exists as a component of palliative care, the setting and role of the care team differs. Hospice programs are far more common than palliative care programs and employ a team of hospice professionals to administer care from the patient's home. Hospice also relies more on the family caregiver and a visiting hospice nurse.

In palliative care programs, the palliative care team is composed of doctors, nurses, and other medical professionals at a facility such as a hospital, extended-care facility, or nursing home where the patient receives quality-of-life treatment. Make sure to provide this type of overview when you explain the function of the multi-disciplinary team and note that each member of the team contributes particular skills and areas of emphasis. Within this interdisciplinary team dynamic, let the patient know that the palliative care physician's area of concentration includes symptom management, as well as continued application of disease-modifying therapy. You also might provide examples of what type of other professionals to expect in the multi-disciplinary team. For example, dyspnea, nausea, weakness, and delirium are all common sources of physical distress among dying patients, so the multi-disciplinary team might include specialists in medical and radiation oncology, anesthesiology, neurology, surgery, and neurosurgery. You also might name some of the advantages of having a multi-disciplinary team, which include decreased unplanned hospital admissions, improved access to health care, enhanced continuity of care, and improved clinical outcome. Helping patients cope and encouraging family involvement with a transition to palliative or hospice care means promoting life at the end of life and helping them see the big picture with respect to what is most important to them. Since family involvement is crucial to hospice care, and families of terminal patients report increased morbidity, mortality, and financial hardship, you also must promote coping strategies for the caregivers who feel helpless and want to give up.

Not all patients are as receptive to discussions about palliative care. Patients who hold out hope for a cure may experience emotions on the extended grief cycle all over again, and you may have to deal with denial as a driving force in their unwillingness to talk about palliative care. As the consulting physician, you may feel that you lack the time required to impart information about palliative care, or you may want to avoid the subject of palliative care because it surrounds the initial conversation with your patient about death and dying. In their book, *Beyond Symptom Management: Physician Roles and Responsibilities in Palliative Care*, Ira Byock, Arthur Caplan, and Lois Snynder note that, "Physicians may be reluctant to refer to palliative care and hospice programs, fearing that patients will interpret the suggestion as abandonment…" However, if you engage in meaningful conversation and explore whatever questions patients and family members may have (i.e. subjective concerns), your patient is less likely to feel that the conversation is a thinly veiled sign of abandonment. Moreover, if you demonstrate knowledge of the support team and talk about why you personally believe the support team you are referring is a good one, the patient is more likely to discuss the transition to palliative care. In cases where the patient seems resistant to the discussion, a number of barriers may be the cause, and your job will be to identify them. Byock, Caplan, and Snyder list a number of common patient/physician barriers to discussing palliative care transition, which include:

- Time limitations
- Medical culture that reinforces denial of death
- Prognostic uncertainty
- Insufficient knowledge
- Ethnic, cultural, and religious challenges
- Legal, regulatory, procedural, or financial barriers
- Education and training deficiencies

So how can you demonstrate that you are referring the patient to a competent group of palliative care specialists? First, it may be helpful to talk about the benefits of psychosocial interventions in reducing distress and improving well-being. Second, you might mention that multi-disciplinary teams share knowledge and are more likely to implement advances in treatment. Third, you might talk about how randomized studies show that inclusion of a nurse in a supportive and informational role is associated with increased patient satisfaction. Finally, you might highlight what you believe to be the characteristics of a well-functioning medical team and provide examples of how the team you recommend meets the criteria. If you do not have a palliative care team to recommend, ask your colleagues to recommend one, or search through an online database. The Center to Advance Palliative Care sponsors a database called Get Palliative Care at **www.getpalliativecare.org/providers**, which provides a state-by-state listing of palliative care services.

# Introducing Families to Palliative or Hospice Care

Educating the patient's family members about what to expect in palliative care is an important part of eliminating uncertainties. It is even more important for gaining consensus to make such a transition, especially among those who must shoulder the burden of care and associated decisions if the patient becomes unable to make autonomous choices near life's end. In their book, *Mastering Communication with Seriously Ill Patients*, Anthony Back *(et al)* provide an eight-step protocol to help the patient and the family construct a big-picture view in terms of their subjective needs for a palliative care transition. You can apply this protocol solely to the patient or in conjunction with the family.

## Step 1

**Prepare yourself.** Give yourself time to think about the case. Consider everything that you have learned about the patient and the patient's family, and formulate what you will say to initiate them into a conversation about palliative care.

## Step 2

**Make sure the family understands the medical situation before you initiate any conversation about palliative care.** Track their emotional data and respond to cues using the techniques outlined in this book.

## Step 3

**Assess their readiness to talk about what is next.** If the patient or any family members appear overwhelmed with emotion, they may need some time and space to gather themselves. An important key to judging emotional readiness stems from their willingness to engage in dialogue. If they appear disengaged, retreat for a while before you reassess their emotional readiness.

## Step 4

**Use big picture questions to elicit a conversation about their subjective values.** Big-picture questions should focus on what is the most valuable, what is most positive, and what they feel makes life precious to them. At this point, you should avoid talking about whether or not these values are feasible; you are simply using this conversation as a staging ground for reassessment of goals. You also should refrain from big-picture questions that elicit conversations about legacy or intimations of death since you want to ease them into a conversation about changing goals. Instead, employ big-picture questions that emphasize the positive and encourage life in the face of impending death. For example, when dealing with a spouse, you might ask what the spouse feels is most important to him or her at this stage. He or she might say, "I'm afraid of being alone if [the spouse] passes." In this case, you might say, "I'm hoping you won't wind up alone either. If the disease progresses into a terminal phase, what would be the most important thing to you right now?" You also might ask another positive big-picture question such as, "What are you hoping for?" If the family member responds with the hope that the patient will get better, ask, "Is there anything else?" Asking these kinds of questions gets family members to think about concerns outside the patient's health, such as their own personal well-being. Once they begin to think about their own subjective desire, you can integrate these values into management and coping strategies, which they might later employ during the palliative care process. You might ask the patient what is going on in their life outside of their medical situation. Getting the patient to talk about their personal life will help you identify their values that exist outside of a hope for a cure. The patient's answer also may indicate the types of coping strategies they use and the effectiveness of those strategies.

## Step 5

**Talk about barriers to decision-making.** A big picture question to ask in this step might be asking what the patient or family feels is the hardest part of the medical problem. This question helps the patient air problems that the patient or family may have been reluctant to discuss until that point. As you facilitate this conversation, you may find that creating dialogue about barriers helps the patient and/or family members work toward a solution that removes them.

## Step 6

**Acknowledge that the current treatments are not working as hoped and offer to make a recommendation.** You can set up the introduction to palliative care by saying that you would like to recommend new treatment options based on what the patient and family said they believe is important. At this point, you can generalize what other people worry about to introduce the goal of pain and symptom control, strengthening relationships, and regaining a sense of control.

## Step 7

**Introduce hospice or palliative care and propose a treatment plan.** This plan should incorporate at least some of the desired goals, and draw honest distinctions between what you believe are long shots and what you believe are reasonable objectives. When talking about hospice or palliative care, refer back to the earlier sections on how to introduce this transition and the five emphasis points of the palliative care setting.

## Step 8

**Ask for feedback on your proposed plan.** If the patient or family shows resistance, demonstrate a willingness to modify your proposal. To find consensus on a treatment plan, repeat steps 4 and 5 until you have a plan everyone can agree with.

# How Patients and Family Members Respond to Transition Discussions

When you approach your patient and the patient's family about transitioning from curative care to palliative care, you can expect to get one of three types of reactions, especially if they begin to realize that you are talking about end-of-life planning. They may accept reality and acquiesce to transition, they may try to negotiate reality and transition, or they may refuse reality and decline a transition. When you reach Step 2 of the eight-step protocol, ask yourself which of these three reactions appear present by reading the verbal and non-verbal cues. Patients and family members who demonstrate acceptance of reality and appear ready for a conversation about a transition to end-of life planning typically ask questions about what happens next rather than dictating what they want to see happen. These patients are ready for end-of-life planning, so you can proceed to eliciting a conversation about their subjective desire using big picture questions.

Patients who try to negotiate reality and any transition you introduce are close to accepting reality and your suggestions, but they want more evidence. You will be able to tell when a patient or family member is trying to negotiate if they raise questions about the assessment and intimate that they want a second opinion. The best way to convince people in this group is to talk in terms of milestones. If you show them the milestones reached along the illness trajectory, they will begin to have a clear understanding of a rapidly declining health pattern. This type of milestone should be presented as hard evidence (e.g. in the form of a scan measuring the growth of lesions over time) and independent of the clinician's opinion. Even if the patient or family member sees the markers, they may want to see further evidence of disease progression from the present to some near point in the future. In such cases, you might suggest continuing therapy for a short trial period using the same methods to track the disease progression.

Patients or family members who refuse reality and decline any transition tend to appear confused, undecided, and removed from the conversation. These people may appear engaged at first when you begin talking but decline to act when the time comes. For example, if you show them the progression of the disease and repeat what you have said when you check for understanding, they may decline to sign a waiver form. In this case, actions speak louder than words. Instead of forcing them to confront the truth, give them more time and provide a safe place to explore their barriers.

# Palliative Care Themes Discussed in Family Meetings

Any family meeting about palliative or hospice care will surround a discussion that touches upon a group of common themes. When you prepare for the family meeting, think about the most common themes that arise in a palliative care conversation and ask yourself which themes you expect to address based on everything you already know about the patient and the patient's family. Remember that advocacy in palliative care does not just involve the patient's needs. You also want to help foster a positive palliative care environment for family members affected by a caregiving, transitional, end-of-life setting. The most common themes you can expect to encounter in a palliative care setting include:

- The nature of the disease and its symptoms
- Prognosis of the patient's illness trajectory
- Information about the medical team
- The emotional demands of caregiving

- The importance of self-care
- How to discuss dying
- How to say goodbye to the patient
- How to manage impending death in hospice care
- The positive aspects of caregiving
- The importance of sharing responsibility of care
- When to seek outside help
- Resource information

# Saying Goodbye to Patients

When you finally discharge your patients into hospice, you probably will never see them again. If you have made the effort to nurture a clinical relationship through two-way communication, it is good form to say goodbye in an appropriate manner. How you say goodbye goes a long way in leaving your patients with a feeling that you genuinely care. It also puts a fitting touch on your commitment in delivering negative medical news in a positive light. If you make the effort to implement all the techniques outlined in this book, but fail to say goodbye to the patient, you risk undoing everything you set out to do by leaving the patient feeling abandoned. From a clinician's perspective, this can be the most awkward part of patient care because the patient probably understands that death is near. In some cases, an official goodbye becomes moot if the patient gets readmitted two weeks later for complications. Nevertheless, you cannot ignore the end of the relationship if your goal is to promote life near the end of life and create a positive effect for the patient entering palliative care. *Mastering Communication with Seriously Ill Patients* offers a seven-step protocol on how to accomplish these objectives.

## Step 1

**Choose an appropriate time and place to say goodbye.** For patients whom you have had a short relationship with, the end of your discussion about transitioning to palliative care may be an appropriate time to say goodbye. For all longstanding clinical relationships, choosing a separate time afterward to say goodbye can have a lasting and powerful effect on the patient's outlook.

## Step 2

**Acknowledge the end of your routine contact.** This sets the stage for a conversation about closure and lets the patient know that the palliative care team will take care of the patient's future medical needs, decisions, appointments, and consultations.

## Step 3

**Invite the patient to respond and use that response as a launching point into a conversation about closure.**

## Step 4

**Frame the goodbye as an appreciation.** For example, you can say something like, "I just want you to know that I've appreciated being your doctor, and I admire your [courage, humor, honesty, directness, etc.]" You also might add a personal touch and tell the patient that you will miss something about them.

## Step 5

**Allow the patient an opportunity to reciprocate the sentiment.** If they reciprocate, respond with an empathic statement. If they say thank you and reciprocate their appreciation, do not minimize this with modesty. For example, instead of saying, "It was nothing; I was just doing my job," you should receive the appreciation appropriately by acknowledging the patient's gratitude and how much your effort means to them.

## Step 6

**Voice your commitment to the patient's ongoing care.** It may take some time for a patient to trust their palliative care team. If so, you might expect to hear from them or their family in the future if they need outside consultation. You can give them this option by saying, "I'm here if you ever need me" or "The palliative care team will keep me informed about everything."

## Step 7

**Reflect on your relationship with the patient after the patient has left your care.** Reflection is an important part of personal and professional growth in the medical profession. Examine the clinical relationship as a whole. Look at what worked, what did not work, and what you have learned from the experience.

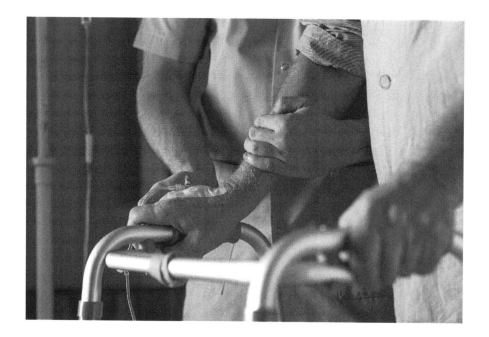

# Chapter 10

# How to Handle End-of-Life Plans and Postmortem Discussions

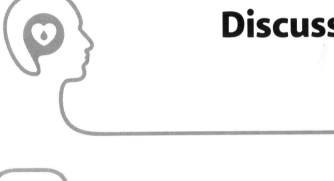

ome patients under consideration for transition to palliative or hospice care may not ask or want to have a conversation about death and dying. For others, you should be ready to talk about it. Conversations about death and dying may include human issues of spirituality, acceptance, setting things right with others, or learning to live during the time that remains. Other conversations about death and dying may include legal aspects and end-of-life-plans such as making a will, consenting to autopsy, organ donation, DNR orders, etc. Conversations with patients about dying can be very awkward and frustrating, or they can be highly rewarding. When patients and family members are in denial of the clinical reality, and you attempt to strip away their defense mechanisms in an abrupt manner instead of gradually working through it, you risk causing hopelessness (an even greater challenge than denial). If you begin to lose hope in the patient, the patient may detect it through verbal or non-verbal communication and lose all remaining hopefor themselves. The best way to initiate a conversation about death and dying is to ask the patient, "Have you thought about what you would want if things do not go as we hope?" Posing death as a possible but still hypothetical question allows for an exploratory dialogue that gets the patient to start thinking about end-of-life plans, even if the patient in denial views them as a contingency. If handled correctly, you should not consider these conversations awkward or burdensome. In fact, many physicians report conversations with patients about death and dying as being "powerful and life changing" to their own experience as well as to the patient's individual outlook of the remaining future. If you follow the steps outlined in this chapter, your conversations with patients will be rewarding instead of frustrating. How you talk about dying may not only make a difference to the patient, but also to your professional and personal life.

# Road Map for End-of-Life Discussion

Before you attempt to talk about end-of-life plans, you should hold a team meeting with your medical staff to discuss the case and reach consensus on important issues involving the legal aspects. Meeting with your medical staff helps to formulate a strategy for discussing end-of-life plans, clarifies roles, and prevents any possibility of sending the patient or family conflicting messages. Depending on the patient and family's acceptance of the clinical reality, you may integrate any conversation about end-of-life plans with your conversation about transition to palliative care, or you may hold them as two separate conversations. For patients or family members who need more time to accept the prognosis, it may be wiser to initiate a conversation about transition to palliative care first since introduction to that topic is more gradual. When the patient reaches the acceptance phase, schedule a pre-conference team meeting, and then schedule an interview with the patient.

When you begin the patient interview, open with introductions and declare your agenda. If you have already conducted a conversation about a transition to palliative care then the patient already knows about the state of the illness and the prescribed treatment goals. Therefore, you can start this conversation by gathering information about the patient's wishes and thoughts regarding death and dying. Since information gathering requires listening, you will find that patients and family members will want to do most of the talking. A 2004 study published by J.R. McDonagh (*et al*) in *Critical Care Medicine* found that family members associated increased listening by the physician with a higher degree of satisfaction in the clinical encounter. You can approach information gathering in three ways. Using the first approach, you could ask the patient directly about his or her thoughts and wishes regarding dying, end-of-life plans, advanced directives, etc. Using the second approach, you could ask the patient to talk about personal experiences with death. If the patient begins talking about specific experiences, ask how these experiences might affect any possible future decisions about end-of of life goals. For patients mentally incapable of making end-of-life plans, you would use the third approach and ask the family or surrogate decision maker what they believe the patient would want if faced with decisions regarding end-of-life plans. When using the third approach, be sure to avoid euphemisms about death. Instead, employ the family meeting techniques outlined in Chapter 7 (ex: circular, strategic or reflexive questioning). As you gather information in your end-of-life discussion, it may help to apply some of the techniques outlined in this book when responding to emotions. You might show empathy, normalize emotional responses, elicit self-expression, repeat the patient's words to demonstrate that you have listened and heard, or praise courage.

After gathering information, make your recommendations about end of life care. If you have already recommended palliative or hospice care, you should discuss legal aspects such as do not resuscitate orders (DNR), autopsy request, organ donation, the living will, etc. However, for the sake of framing negative medical news in a positive light, you should always ask the patient if he or she would like to talk about the human aspects of death and dying (spirituality, acceptance, etc.) before talking about the legal aspects of end-of-life plans. When you make your recommendation, use the shared decision-making approach to ease the burden of responsibility. Give the patient or surrogate decision maker the option of delaying these decisions, particularly if they feel they need to talk it over with anyone else who these plans would affect. Finally, show praise and support for the decisions (if made) and reassure the patient and/or family members that you will continue to offer your council, and that you will do everything possible to make sure that the patient lives comfortably through the process. To show support for a decision, you might say something like, "This is a tough situation, but I think that we are making the most reasonable decision given the options that are available." Using "we" in this statement instead of "you" reaffirms the notion of a joint decision and helps ease the burden of responsibility for family members who might feel isolated in the decisions they face in an end-of-life scenario. When you finalize the agreed-upon end-of-life plans, summarize the plan along with any directives, offer assistance to high priority issues such as symptom management or spiritual needs, ask for feedback, and schedule a follow-up meeting.

## Common Mistakes in an End-of-Life Discussion

If you are someone who needs to practice this type of communication, seek training from a program that offers role-playing scenarios. Communication training can help you learn to explore alternate ways of looking at the dilemmas of dying patients. Poor communication during the end-of-life process can result in loss of clinical confidence, inefficient decisions, or avoidance of critical mental or physical health issues. For example, if you express sadness because you believe you cannot do anything more for the patient or if the patient reminds you of your own previous losses, you may wind up avoiding the patient by sending a member of the junior staff to deal with your responsibilities. The best way to approach end-of-life communication is to know what *not* to do.

## Mistake 1

**Telling the patient there is nothing more you can do.** This statement carries the assumption that no further medical care will amount to anything, including a shift in goals of care. If you say this to a patient, they may think that also includes any transition to palliative care, particularly if they do not fully understand the goals of palliative care (including treatment changes). Knowledge deficits, whether on the part of the physician or the patient, can create unintended resistance to your medical recommendations for end-of-life care. Instead, be more specific and tell the patient that although the disease has advanced beyond curing, there are ways to improve the quality of life.

## Mistake 2

**Placing the responsibility of decisions on the patient rather than framing it as a shared decision.** For example, if you ask a patient what he or she would like to do in the event of a cardiac arrest, you place a DNR responsibility on the patient, which contradicts your commitment to shared decision-making.

## Mistake 3

**Causing the patient to associate certain goals of palliative care with curative therapy.** For example, if you tell the patient that he or she needs to gain more weight in order to receive more chemotherapy, the patient may think that gaining weight is more important than the goal of improving quality of life. At this point, chemotherapy may serve no purpose, and the patient may blame his or her own efforts if weight loss continues. Instead, you should explain why the patient probably will not be able to meet any of the goals of curative therapy and why the patient will be able to meet the goals of palliative care.

## Mistake 4

**Saying the disease has "advanced" or "progressed" to announce that the patient is dying.** While you may use these words as euphemisms for a worsening condition along the illness trajectory, you should try to avoid euphemisms in the dying phase. Instead, be frank with your patient and tell them that he or she has entered the terminal phase of the illness.

## Mistake 5

**Telling the patient that his or her body has failed to respond to treatments.** Phrasing treatment failure in such a way appears to blame the patient. Instead, place the blame elsewhere and tell the patient that the treatments did not work.

**Mistake 6**

**Using graphic descriptions to explain DNR directives or any medical procedure.** Describing things in this way accomplishes nothing other than traumatizing the patient and leaving them unable to make a decision. For example, if you believe that CPR would not save your patient, and you describe all the unpleasant things about administering CPR, you would be attempting to manipulate the patient's decision through coercion. Instead, explain why a procedure will not extend life or why it would prolong the patient's suffering.

**Mistake 7**

**Labeling the patient. This sets up the patient as an adversary to you and to everyone involved in the palliative care process.** It diminishes trust in the patient-doctor relationship and complicates shared decision-making. Instead, engage the patient's problem and give it a chance to evolve over time. If nothing changes, at least you gave the patient an opportunity to change under the best possible conditions.

# Discussing Human Issues about the End-of-Life

While some researchers suggest that doctors should not depart from their area of expertise to promote a non-medical agenda, studies show that spiritual involvement positively correlates with health behaviors, medical compliance, and coping with illness. As the aphorism goes, the primary task of the physician is to "cure sometimes, relieve often, and comfort always." In response to skepticism of spirituality's effectiveness in palliative care, Koenig, Idler, and Kasl conducted a systematic review of more than 1200 studies on the religion-health relationship and published their findings in the *International Journal of Psychiatry in Medicine*. Their review covered cases conducted by different investigators, different health facilities, and diverse populations across the United States recorded over the span of a century. According to Koenig (*et al*), "The vast majority of these studies show a relationship between greater religious involvement, better mental health, better physical health, and lower use of health services." Only recently have palliative care practitioners begun to recognize the importance of treating spiritual and existential suffering in the end-of-life process by developing interventions and establishing spirituality as a priority.

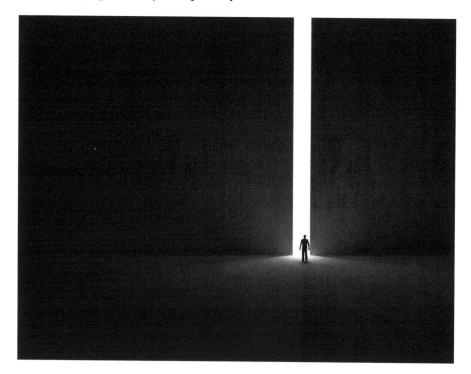

Patients may raise the topic of death in different ways. For example, if your patient raises questions about assisted suicide or euthanasia, you should not feel as if the patient is challenging your ethical boundaries. Asking such questions may be their own way of trying to test your willingness to talk about death and to understand what the dying process is like. If you respond with openness about the topic of death and avoid taking a defensive position, it may restore the patient's sense of certainty and hope in what lies ahead. If the patient presses you on the issue of assisted suicide or euthanasia, keep the emphasis on affective palliative treatments that reduce suffering and try to steer the conversation toward a discussion about human issues involving the dying process, such as spirituality. Whether the patient alludes to their desire to talk about spirituality or you direct the patient toward this topic, you might consider using an open-ended question to get the conversation started. For example, you might say, "Are there any religious or spiritual concerns you think we should talk about?" Since you cannot offer answers to these larger questions, it is best to listen to what the patient has to say and reflect their own words back at them in the form of a question to continue their elaboration of existential and spiritual concern. For example, if a patient says, "I don't feel like the person I used to be," you might reflect this as a question by asking, "Who do you feel that you used to be?"

# Spirituality and Existential Anxiety

Sogyal Rinpoche, author of the *Tibetan Book of Living and Dying*, once wrote that all religions stress the power of forgiveness. Through forgiveness, we purify ourselves from our past mistakes and prepare ourselves more completely for the journey through death. The struggle that patients experience near the end of their life is the conflict between spirituality and existential anxiety. Dr. Christina Puchalski, who designed the spirituality assessment FICA (faith, importance, community, and address) defines spirituality as "that which allows a person to experience transcendent meaning in life." Psychotherapist Emmy van Deurzen defines existential anxiety as "that basic unease which we experience as soon as we become self-conscious and aware of our vulnerability and possible death… It is a measure of the extent to which we face up to the basic question of whether we will be or not be." Likewise, Eric Ettema (*et al*) defines existential anxiety as feeling hopeless, burdening others, losing a sense of dignity and the will to live, having a desire for death, or having one's sense of identity come under threat. Existential loneliness also has entered the literature, which Ettema defines as "an intolerable emptiness, sadness, and longing that results from the awareness of one's fundamental separateness as a human being."The question anguishing most terminal patients is the uncertainty of what lies at the end of the road, if anything. Does existence transcend or cease upon biological death? Is there any meaning to this life? Was it wasted? Are there any regrets? Is there unfinished business? Existential suffering in the face of death demands the examination of all the events that define an entire lifetime, but for which there are no clear answers or knowable future. In order to help the patient talk about their spiritual concerns and/or existential anxiety, consider using Pulchaski's FICA assessment to obtain the patient's spiritual history by asking the questions provided in Table 4.

*Table 4. Pulchaski's FICA Assessment of Spiritual History*

| F | Faiths or beliefs |
|---|---|
| | • What is your faith or belief? |
| | • Do you consider yourself spiritual or religious? |
| | • What things do you believe in that give meaning to life? |
| **I** | **Importance and influence** |
| | • Is it important to your life? |
| | • What influence does it have on how you take care of yourself? |

| | |
|---|---|
| | • How have your beliefs influenced your behavior during this illness? |
| **C** | **Community** |
| | • Are you part of a spiritual or religious community? |
| | • Is this of support to you, and how? |
| | • Is there a person or group of people whom you really love or who are really important to you? |
| **A** | **Address** |
| | • How would you like me, your health care provider, to address these issues in health care? |

Exploring the patient's spiritual history will begin to open a dialogue that can translate into a form of existential therapy. The goal of this kind of therapy is to talk about the shared experience of life. Within this shared experience is our capacity for self-awareness, our freedoms and responsibilities, the need for others, the search for meaning, the anxiety of living, and the awareness of death and possible non-being. The best way to discuss these issues is to ask questions, listen, and share some of your own experiences as they relate to the patient's concerns. Perhaps you might share stories about how other patients faced death and dying. The key to existential therapy is not to have an answer to these questions and concerns, but to provide the patient with a sense of feeling heard and being part of a shared experience. In their book, *Psychotherapeutic Interventions at the End of Life: A Focus on Meaning and Spirituality*, Breitbart *(et al)* note, "The value of existential psychotherapy in end-of-life care is that it encourages patients to seriously explore their past, present, and future in terms of meaningful choices and the experiences that created and continue to generate their story. By challenging the notions of heightened awareness, personal freedom, and responsibility, patients begin to meaningfully reflect upon and take ownership of the lives they have chosen, and of the possibilities that are still available until the moment of their death." Helping patients explore the "why" of their existence and the meaning of their lives offers a way to bear the burden of suffering and eventual death with strength and dignity.

# Discussing Legal Issues about the End-of-Life

Preparing for death requires more than just psychological and spiritual therapy. If you are part of a palliative care team, you will have to broach the subject of your legal responsibilities during and after the patient's death. Legal matters are the last thing that most patients want to discuss as they enter the terminal phase of illness. Nevertheless, the patient and the patient's family need to have their affairs in order ahead of time. The easiest way to accomplish this is to ask the patient or family members if they have any specific administrative concerns, such as a living will, that you need to address. If the patient or family members do not appear ready to discuss death, you can frame the living will issue in terms of hoping for the best and planning for the worst, and proceed to ask questions about directives. As the health care practitioner, you will have to achieve informed consent regarding any possible legal issues that require near-death or postmortem intervention, including:

- CPR as symptomatic relief
- DNR orders
- Request for autopsy
- Organ donation
- Requests to die sooner
- Requests to withdraw from life support or life-sustaining treatments

Dying is a highly emotional experience. To reiterate, you should not use legal issues such as DNR orders or requests for autopsy as a means of introducing dying. Patients will feel vulnerable, distracted, and terrified. If you start talking about chest compressions or intubation, they may sign off on a directive without realizing or intending to. Since obtaining DNR orders follows the process of informed consent, you risk ethically violating autonomy by handling legal issues about death and dying before giving the patient a chance to explore spiritual concerns and existential anxieties. However, medical institutions recently have begun to re-examine the nature of DNR. While doctors view CPR as a futile therapy, patients continue to hold widespread illusions about CPR as life extension in the face of immanent death. Due to this disconnect between doctors and patients, many institutions around the world no longer require their medical staff to discuss the directive. Doctors now discuss CPR as an intervention as long as an understanding exists that symptomatic relief is the goal of the palliative care staff as opposed to life extension. That said, studies show that roughly one-third of dying patients agree to CPR when offered. Therefore, most of your discussion about end-of-life legal issues should focus on the objectives of treatment. If you discuss DNR with your patients, focus your discussion on educating the patient about the nature of DNR and its objectives. Be sure to mention that any directive can be changed at any time if the patient so chooses. While consensus about DNR has changed over the years, some institutions still require discussion of a DNR directive that obtains informed consent. Before having a conversation about DNR, know if your institution requires an informed consent type of discussion. Become familiar with local DNR laws and relevant forms to improve the technical aspects of your communication with the patient. If a health care agent tries to override a DNR directive signed by a patient, it is your responsibility is to explain how the local laws aim to preserve patient autonomy. Education of DNR should include information about:

- Prognosis
- Treatment alternatives
- The low efficacy of CPR
- The human cost of inefficacious treatments at the end of life
- Your clear opinion about the DNR directives based on clinical data

Some directives, such as autopsy and organ donation, may involve getting informed consent of someone other than the patient. Making requests for organ donations and autopsies are also among the more uncomfortable end-of-life discussions doctors face, particularly if you have just informed a family member about the death of a loved one. Family members in a high emotional state are more likely to refuse such requests. To facilitate these discussions, consider using the CONES approach outlined in Chapter 4, but realize that however you choose to discuss the matter, your main legal responsibility with respect to autopsy and organ donation is to keep the administrative steps simple and with no effort from next of kin. Relatives do not want to feel bothered by these directives, so you should not use the CONES approach to press them into saying yes.

Another advanced directive you need to cover is the request to withdraw life support or life-sustaining treatment should the hospital admit your palliated patient into an intensive care unit. Most deaths in intensive care units occur *after* decisions to limit or withdraw life support, which makes this advanced directive an important topic for discussion. Researchers argue that life support withdrawal plays a critical role in palliative care because certain directives may cause inadequate pain management. In order to make an informed decision about an advanced directive, the patient needs to know which withdrawals may cause suffering or discomfort, especially since the goal of palliative care is to reduce suffering. For example, the withdrawal of mechanical ventilation is one of the few life-sustaining treatments where withdrawal can cause discomfort. Therefore, to gain informed consent, your discussion about this advanced directive should not only include *whether* to withdraw life support, but to educate the patient about *how* life support is withdrawn. In order to execute an advanced directive about withdrawing life support, you must:

- Recognize that the patient or surrogate decision maker needs informed consent
- Take steps to obtain informed consent
- Provide your recommendations and link them to the values cited by the patient
- Respect the right of patients or their surrogates to make decisions about the process
- Develop and communicate an explicit plan for carrying out the procedure and dealing with complications
- Document the plan and the patient's consent in the medical record

To educate the patient about withdrawal of life support, start by talking about which procedures will cause discomfort or suffering and which will not. Next, talk about the ethical principles that medical staffers are bound to observe. For example, you could explain that any withdrawal of life support is considered a medical procedure, and it is ethical to remove treatments that are no longer desired or do not provide the patient comfort. However, the patient should be aware that any withdrawal intended to hasten death is morally and legally problematic. In his medical journal, *Principles and Practice of Withdrawing Life-Sustaining Treatments*, Gordon Rubenfeld writes, "Ethical and clinical principles should guide optimal management of some aspects of withdrawing life-sustaining treatment... [However], ethicists draw a line between withdrawing life-sustaining treatments when the expected but unintended effect is to hasten death and providing a treatment with the sole intent of hastening death."

When terminal patients make a request to die sooner, you should avoid saying that euthanasia is illegal or not in your practice. Instead, try to explore these statements in an empathic manner. Such requests may represent signs of existential anxiety in low ebb, which may later fluctuate to a higher pitch. Moreover, a request do die sooner may reflect feelings of demoralization, depression, suicidal ideation, or poorly controlled pain management — all of which can be treated if recognized. To explore these requests in an empathic manner, respond by saying something like, "I'd like to hear more about your desire for me to help you die." For further reading on the legal and ethical aspects of life-support withdrawal, *Principles of Critical Care* by Jesse Hall *(et al)* covers the topic in greater depth.

# Communicating to Promote Life near the End of Life

Your final task in presenting negative medical news in a positive light is to encourage the patient to continue living a productive, meaningful life near the end of life, if possible. You might start by revisiting any personal issues that you recorded in the patient's medical history and assessing if the patient has maintained or regained a sense of meaning and purpose in the final stretch of life. Sometimes this means challenging patients to do something they always put off doing; in other cases, it might mean making peace with past mistakes or old regrets. In their book, *A Physician's Guide to End-of-Life Care*, Byock, Caplan, and Snyder state that "Although a number of valuable opportunities exist during the time of living identified as 'dying,' they are just that — opportunities. However, assessments must not become criteria for judging a patient or family's worth. Some issues of personal and family history will not lend themselves to forgiveness, and extremely difficult clinical or social situations may afford no chance for introspection or the intimate communication required for reconciliation. Sudden death, critical care settings, severe, uncontrolled symptoms, serious family dysfunction, social circumstances, poverty, or psychosocial problems all represent significant challenges to a satisfying sense of life closure." To this end, you must avoid losing hope for the patient, as this can undermine opportunities to promote life near the end of life.

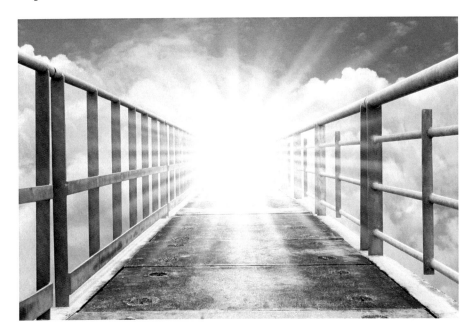

The best way to lift a patient out of hopelessness is to help the patient create a new goal. In Chapter 5, we defined this type of goal as a displacement behavior, which can take the form of a hobby, an artistic creation, or an intellectual endeavor. A displacement goal might be a previously held ambition that was never fulfilled, or it can be used as a way of healing past regrets. In order to find the displacement goal, begin exploring sources of hope for the patient. Along the way, identify any potential obstacles that might present themselves in the pursuit of this goal. If the patient has trouble naming sources of hope, ask the patient to recall uplifting memories. Encourage them to remember the good things they have done in their life, and to feel positive about the way they have lived.

Focus on their successes and virtues, not on their failings. Keep in mind that the most common obstacle to finding an appropriate displacement behavior is the unrelenting pain that prevents the patient from reaching the stated goal. In the book, *Preparing for Death and Helping the Dying*, Sangye Khadro notes that some patients need to forgive themselves for past actions. As a physician, you can help them to do this by "encouraging them to express their heartfelt regret for their mistakes and ask for forgiveness. Remind them that past actions are over and cannot be changed, so it is best to let go of them. If the person truly regrets making mistakes and wishes to [change], there is no reason they cannot find forgiveness. If there are specific people the person has harmed, encourage the person to seek the person out, express regret, and request forgiveness."

Dying patients tend to focus on statistics and averages when they learn that they have entered the final phase of an illness. Constant focus on how much time remains causes constant worry and prevents the patient from living in the moment or looking forward. You can help patients find hope in their tomorrow by getting them to focus on the next visit from a loved one or something that provides positive anticipation. According to a study published in the *Archives of Internal Medicine*, patients with advanced cancer who avoided hospitalizations and life-prolonging measures, accepted frequent visits by a pastor or chaplain, and maintained a therapeutic alliance with their oncologist had the highest reported quality of life at the end of their life. You also might suggest engaging the patient in a new type of therapy introduced by Harvey Chochinov at the University of Manitoba called "dignity therapy."

Chochinov's therapy uses a trained therapist who presents a series of questions to the patient about his or her life and the parts or events they believe were the most important to them. The therapist writes down the answers and compiles the narrative into a printed document. This may sound somewhat similar to a will, but with a difference in content. A will acts as a living testimony to the patient's legal desires, dignity therapy acts as a living testimony to the life of the patient — their thoughts, emotions, experiences, trials, and triumphs, as seen through their own eyes. Telling one's life story in printed form can be highly therapeutic and in many ways, the printed testimony serves as a way to live on after the moment of passing. Patients formerly enrolled in dignity therapy have told life stories as long as fifty pages. Some patients even revised the memories of their lives, remembering only positive things or reinterpreting events according to perception. Some patients even used their stories to apologize for mistakes they had made. According to Chochinov, one alcoholic patient told his life story so that his grandchildren would choose a different path. Being of service to others and helping the living as well as the dying is one way this kind of therapy can help your dying patients find meaning and purpose in their own lives.

## CASE STUDY

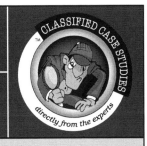

Name: Dr. Christina Puchalski
Title: Internist and Geriatrician
District: Washington D.C.

I see spirituality as that which allows a person to experience transcendent meaning in life. Patients may express this as a relationship with God, but it can also be about nature, art, music, family, or community — whatever beliefs and values give a person a sense of meaning and purpose in life. A spiritual history is a beliefs or values history that explicitly opens the door to a conversation about the role of spirituality and religion in the person's life. This conversation is extremely important for patients who are gravely ill and for dying patients. Spiritual questions that come up for these patients include: What gives my life meaning? Why is this thing happening to me? How will I survive this loss? What will happen to me when life ends?

We, as clinicians, do not know the answers, but I do see it as our role to support and encourage people as they search for their own answers to these questions. Their spiritual beliefs, religious faith, and values are resources, and it is important to see this work as a team effort and to refer patients to chaplains and spiritual directors as needed. Patients learn to cope with and understand their suffering through their spiritual beliefs, or the spiritual dimension of their lives. It is through that dimension that I think the compassionate, caring part of the doctor/patient relationship becomes important. We do not normally think of it that way, but to me, it's a very spiritual interaction. Physicians work in a service profession. Our job is caring for people; I think that in and of itself is spiritual work.

What has happened over the last 30 years is that science has really led medicine, [causing neglect] to the non-technical aspects of medicine. The spiritual assessment reclaims or brings us back to those compassionate, caregiving roots of the patient-doctor relationship. I see a spiritual assessment as an opportunity for physicians, nurses, or other health care practitioners to start discussing these spiritual issues, which are so important with patients. Doing the spiritual history also helps health care providers understand the role that spirituality plays in the patient-clinician relationship itself.

Those things will probably not come out in a typical medical interview, and yet we are seeing from a number of surveys that spiritual issues are very important to many people. Oftentimes they need permission to talk about those kinds of issues. Without some signal from the physician, patients may feel that these topics are not appropriate or welcome. When you get involved in a discussion with a patient about his or her spirituality, you enter the domain of what gives that person meaning and purpose. When you begin to find out about why the person is suffering, and to listen to that person, you cannot help but notice a change in the quality of the relationship. Physicians who have incorporated the spiritual assessment write back and tell me about it. They say that the nature of the patient-doctor relationship changes — as soon as they bring up these questions, they feel that it establishes a certain level of intimacy in terms of really understanding who that person is at a much deeper level than they are accustomed to. The relationship feels less superficial.

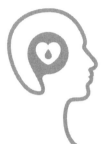

# Conclusion

ur hope in writing this book is that you have come away with a better understanding of what it takes to present negative medical news in a positive light. If you started with the assumption that patient-doctor communication was not a part of your job, you are certainly wiser now. A good communicator uses many methods to foster cooperation and increase patient satisfaction in managed care. As you continue to practice the techniques outlined in this book, you will gain experience and become the kind of health care practitioner that patients can trust. When others fail to communicate, that is where you come in. You will be a master of nuance, entrusted to help others, and use your expertise to the best of your ability. The way the medical profession practices medicine may change over time, but its changes will always create new opportunities for you to make a difference in the lives of others. The road ahead is both challenging and rewarding. We wish you luck.

Before closing this book and heading off to employ these techniques, examine the questions at the end of this conclusion, as they will help you determine just how ready you are to communicate with your patients. If the key to professional happiness is a subjective reality, perhaps the key to yours is in being of service to others. As author and physician Swami Sivananda once said, "Put your heart, mind, intellect, and soul into even your smallest acts. This is the secret of success."

## Questions to Ask After Reading this Book

a. Do I have a better understanding of my patient's emotional needs?

b. Do I feel comfortable using the strategies and protocols outlined in this book?

c. Do I feel it is feasible to support the patient in the manners described?

d. Do I feel these strategies will save time, eliminate misunderstanding, reduce conflicts, and satisfy both patient and physician objectives?

e. Is there any information I am unsure about?

f. Where can I find information (in this book or otherwise) that will lead me to my answer?

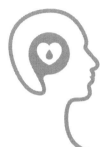

# Resources

## Informational Resources on Palliative Care

- American Association of Retired Persons (AARP) (end of life, wills, estate planning, etc.): **www.aarp.org/families/end_life**

- American Academy of Hospice and Palliative Medicine: **www.aahpm.org**

- Palliative care nursing: **www.palliativecarenursing.net**

## Palliative Care Training Programs

- **ACP-ASIM End-of-Life Care Patient Education Project.** Educational materials developed by a working group of physicians and patient advocates to facilitate conversations among physicians, patients, and their families

- **Association for Death Education and Counseling (ADEC).** One of the oldest multidisciplinary professional organizations in the field of dying, death, and bereavement

- **Educating Future Physicians in Palliative and End-of-Life Care (EFPPEC).** Palliative and end-of-life care education for undergraduate medical students and clinical postgraduate trainees at Canada's seventeen Medical Schools

- **End of Life Physician Education Resource Center (EPERC).** End of Life Physician Education Resource Center for educational materials about end of life issues. Assists physician educators in locating high-quality, peer-reviewed training materials

- **The EPEC Project.** Program designed to educate all physicians on the essential clinical competencies required to provide quality end-of-life care

- **Harvard Medical School Program in Palliative Care Education and Practice.** Offers physicians and nurses intensive learning in the clinical practice and teaching of interdisciplinary palliative care, as well as leading improvements in practice at their own institutions

- **Hospice Education Institute.** Serves individuals and organizations interested in improving and expanding hospice and palliative care throughout the United States and around the world

- **The Institute for Palliative Medicine at San Diego Hospice.** One of the largest hospice and palliative care programs in the United States. The one-year Palliative Medicine Fellowship Program is the largest palliative medicine fellowship program in North America, and includes international programs

- **University of Washington Center for Palliative Care Education.** Educational resource center and training program designed to improve palliative care for people with HIV/AIDS

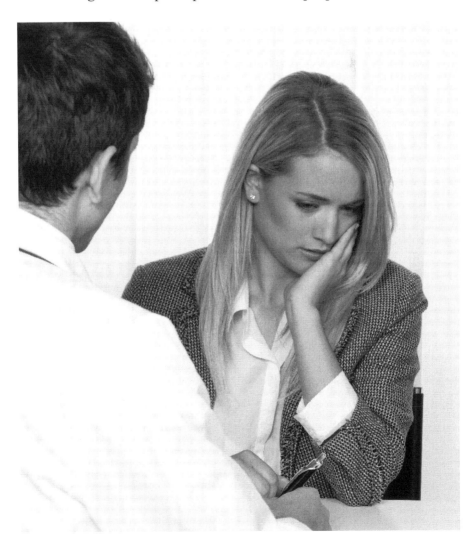

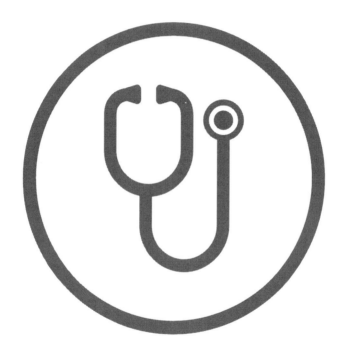

# The Four
# Habits Model
# Full Version

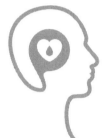

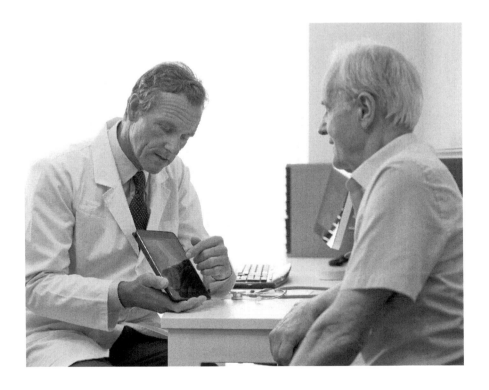

# The Four Habits Model

| Habit | Skills | Techniques and Examples | Payoff |
|---|---|---|---|
| **INVEST IN THE BEGINNING** | Create rapport quickly | • Introduce self to everyone in the room<br>• Acknowledge wait<br>• Convey knowledge of patient's history by commenting on prior visit or problem<br>• Attend to patient's comfort<br>• Make a social comment or ask a nonmedical question to put patient at ease<br>• Adapt own language, pace, and posture in response to patient | • Establishes a welcoming atmosphere<br>• Allows faster access to real reason for visit<br>• Increases diagnostic accuracy<br>• Requires less work<br>• Minimizes "Oh, by the way ... " at the end of visit<br>• Facilitates negotiating an agenda<br>• Decreases potential for conflict |
| | Elicit patient's concerns | • Start with open-ended questions:<br>– "What would you like help with today?"<br>Or, "I understand that you're here for ... Could you tell me more about that?"<br>– "What else?"<br>• Speak directly with patient when using an interpreter | |
| | Plan the visit with the patient | • Repeat concerns back to check understanding<br>• Let patient know what to expect: "How about if we start with talking more about ..., then I'll do an exam, and then we'll go over possible tests/ways to treat this? Sound OK?"<br>• Prioritize when necessary: "Let's make sure we talk about X and Y. It sounds like you also want to make sure we cover Z. If we can't get to the other concerns, let's ... " | |
| **ELICIT THE PATIENT'S PERSPECTIVE** | Ask for patient's ideas | • Assess patient's point of view:<br>– "What do you think is causing your symptoms?"<br>– "What worries you most about this problem?"<br>• Ask about ideas from significant others | • Respects diversity<br>• Allows patient to provide important diagnostic clues<br>• Uncovers hidden concerns<br>• Reveals use of alternative treatments or requests for tests<br>• Improves diagnosis of depression and anxiety |
| | Elicit specific requests | • Determine patient's goal in seeking care: "When you've been thinking about this visit, how were you hoping I could help?" | |
| | Explore the impact on the patient's life | • Check context: "How has the illness affected your daily activities/work/family?" | |
| **DEMONSTRATE EMPATHY** | Be open to patient's emotions | • Assess changes in body language and voice tone<br>• Look for opportunities to use brief empathic comments or gestures | • Adds depth and meaning to the visit<br>• Builds trust, leading to better diagnostic information, adherence, and outcomes<br>• Makes limit-setting or saying "no" easier |
| | Make at least one empathic statement | • Name a likely emotion: "That sounds really upsetting."<br>• Compliment patient on efforts to address problem | |
| | Convey empathy nonverbally | • Use a pause, touch, or facial expression | |
| | Be aware of your own reactions | • Use own emotional response as a clue to what patient might be feeling<br>• Take a brief break if necessary | |
| **INVEST IN THE END** | Deliver diagnostic information | • Frame diagnosis in terms of patient's original concerns<br>• Test patient's comprehension | • Increases potential for collaboration<br>• Influences health outcomes<br>• Improves adherence<br>• Reduces return calls and visits<br>• Encourages self care |
| | Provide education | • Explain rationale for tests and treatments<br>• Review possible side effects and expected course of recovery<br>• Recommend lifestyle changes<br>• Provide written materials and refer to other resources | |
| | Involve patient in making decisions | • Discuss treatment goals<br>• Explore options, listening for the patient's preferences<br>• Set limits respectfully: "I can understand how getting that test makes sense to you. From my point of view, since the results won't help us diagnose or treat your symptoms, I suggest we consider this instead."<br>• Assess patient's ability and motivation to carry out plan | |
| | Complete the visit | • Ask for additional questions: "What questions do you have?"<br>• Assess satisfaction: "Did you get what you needed?"<br>• Reassure patient of ongoing care | |

©Physician Education & Development, TPMG, Inc. No relation to Stephen R. Covey's book, *The 7 Habits of Highly Effective People*

# The SEGUE Framework Checklist

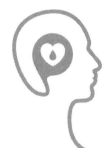

| Patient: | Fellow/Resident: | | | |
|---|---|---|---|---|
| **Set the Stage** | | Yes | No | NA |
| 1. Establishes rapport | | | | |
| 2. Maintains patient's privacy (e.g. closes door) | | | | |
| 3. Describes clinician's reason or agenda for the visit | | | | |
| 4. Maintains a respectful attitude and tone | | | | |
| 5. Makes a personal connection during visit (e.g. goes beyond medical issues at hand) | | | | |

| Elicit Information | Yes | No | NA |
|---|---|---|---|
| 6. Assesses patient's/family's understanding of illness | | | |
| 7. Explores and clarifies key physical symptoms and their treatment | | | |
| 8. Explores and clarifies key psychosocial issues and concerns, and how they have been managed | | | |
| 9. Assesses spiritual/existential issues and concerns | | | |
| 10. Checks/clarifies information (e.g. summarizes, asks follow-up questions) | | | |
| 11. Obtains a thorough past medical history | | | |
| 12. Elicits concerns and worries | | | |
| 13. Determines how health problems affect the patient's daily living, functional status, and quality of life | | | |
| 14. Generally avoids directive and/or leading questions, especially early in the interview | | | |
| 15. Gives pt/family opportunity/time to talk (e.g. listens carefully, does not interrupt) | | | |
| 16. Gives patient/family undivided attention (e.g. sits down, faces patient, acknowledges comments) | | | |

| Give Information | Yes | No | NA |
|---|---|---|---|
| 17. Assesses patient's/family's desire for information and how information should be shared | | | |
| 18. Explains rationale for current diagnostic and treatment plans | | | |
| 19. Teaches patient about his/her medical condition and the diagnostic and treatment options, (e.g. provides feedback/education about diagnosis, current status, management, exams and testing) | | | |
| 20. Educates and supports patient/family about end-of-life issues (e.g. pain and symptom management, prognosis, nutrition/hydration, hospice care, active dying) | | | |
| 21. Encourages patient/family to ask questions | | | |
| 22. Communicates information to patient/family based on their level of understanding (e.g. avoids/ jargon) | | | |
| **Understand the Patient's/ Family's Perspective** | **Yes** | **No** | **NA** |
| 23. Elicits and responds to patient values, goals, and preferences about managing the illness | | | |

| | | | |
|---|---|---|---|
| 24. Explores how family is coping with the illness, including family burden | | | |
| 25. Negotiates goals of treatment | | | |
| 26. Mediates conflicts (e.g. intra-family, between clinicians and patient) | | | |
| **Respond to Emotions** | **Yes** | **No** | **NA** |
| 27. Acknowledges patient's accomplishments/progress/challenges | | | |
| 28. Recognizes and acknowledges affect | | | |
| 29. Deepens the encounter by appropriately eliciting, exploring, and responding to affect | | | |
| 30. Avoids changing the subject and/or giving information in response to emotion | | | |
| 31. Employs empathic verbal behaviors in an appropriate and effective manner (e.g. acknowledging affect, naming, normalization, reflection) | | | |
| 32. Employs facilitating verbal behaviors in an appropriate and effective manner (e.g. attentive listening, silence, open posture) | | | |
| 33. Employs empathic and facilitating non-verbal behaviors in an effective and appropriate manner (e.g. maintain eye contact, touch, facial expression, head nodding) | | | |

| End the Encounter | Yes | No | NA |
|---|---|---|---|
| 34. Asks if there is anything else patient would like to discuss | | | |
| 35. Reviews next steps with patient including plans for follow-up | | | |
| Comments: | | | |

| Visit Date: | Review Date: | Reviewer: |
|---|---|---|

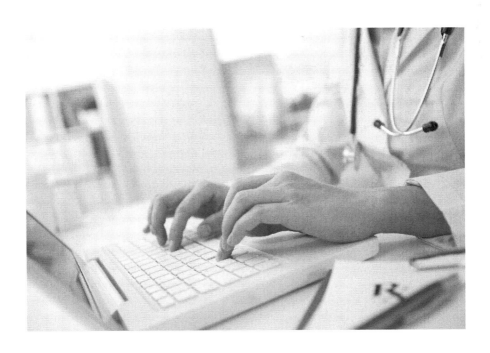

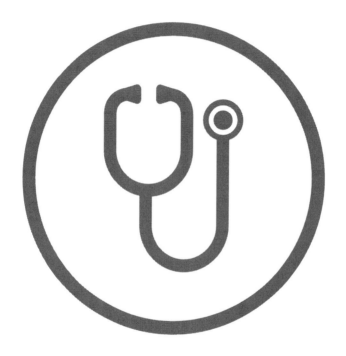

# Calgary-Cambridge Guide

## INITIATING THE SESSION

### Establishing initial rapport

1. **Greets** patient and obtains patient's name

2. **Introduces** self, role, and nature of interview; obtains consent if necessary

3. **Demonstrates respect** and interest, attends to patient's physical comfort

## Identifying the reason(s) for the consultation

4. **Identifies** the **patient's problems** or the issues that the patient wishes to address with appropriate **opening question** (e.g. "What problems brought you to the hospital?" or "What would you like to discuss today?" or "What questions did you hope to get answered today?")

5. **Listens** attentively to the patient's opening statement, without interrupting or directing patient's response

6. **Confirms list and screens** for further problems (e.g. "so that's headaches and tiredness, anything else?")

7. **Negotiates agenda** taking both patient's and physician's needs into account

# GATHERING INFORMATION

## Exploration of patient's problems

8. **Encourages patient to tell the story** of the problem(s) from when first started to the present in own words (clarifying reason for presenting now)

9. **Uses open and closed questioning techniques**, appropriately moving from open to closed

10. **Listens** attentively, allowing patient to complete statements without interruption and leaving space for patient to think before answering or go on after pausing

11. **Facilitates** patient's responses verbally and non–verbally e.g. use of encouragement, silence, repetition, paraphrasing, interpretation

12. **Picks up** verbal and non–verbal **cues** (body language, speech, facial expression, affect); **checks out and acknowledges** as appropriate

13. **Clarifies** patient's statements that are unclear or need amplification (e.g. "Could you explain what you mean by light headed?")

14. Periodically **summarizes** to verify own understanding of what the patient has said; invites patient to correct interpretation or provide further information.

15. **Uses** concise, **easily understood questions and comments**, avoids or adequately explains jargon

16. Establishes dates and sequence of events

### Additional skills for understanding the patient's perspective

17. Actively determines and appropriately explores:

- patient's **ideas** (i.e. beliefs re cause)
- patient's **concerns** (i.e. worries) regarding each problem
- patient's **expectations**: (i.e. goals, what help the patient had expected for each problem)
- effects: how each problem **affects** the patient's life

18. Encourages patient to express feelings

# PROVIDING STRUCTURE TO THE CONSULTATION

## Making organization overt

19. **Summarizes** at the end of a specific line of inquiry to confirm understanding before moving on to the next section

20. Progresses from one section to another using **signposting, transitional statements**; includes rationale for next section

### Attending to flow

21. Structures interview in logical **sequence**

22. Attends to **timing** and keeping interview on task

# BUILDING RELATIONSHIP

### Using appropriate nonverbal behavior

23. Demonstrates appropriate nonverbal behavior

- eye contact, facial expression
- posture, position, and movement
- vocal cues e.g. rate, volume, intonation

24. If reads, writes notes, or uses computer, does in a manner that does not interfere with dialogue or rapport

25. Demonstrates appropriate confidence

### Developing rapport

26. **Accepts** legitimacy of patient's views and feelings; **is not judgmental**

27. **Uses empathy** to communicate understanding and appreciation of the patient's feelings or predicament, overtly **acknowledges patient's views and feelings**

28. **Provides support**: expresses concern, understanding, willingness to help; acknowledges coping efforts and appropriate self-care; offers partnership

29. **Deals sensitively** with embarrassing and disturbing topics and physical pain, including when associated with physical examination

### Involving the patient

30. **Shares thinking** with patient to encourage patient's involvement (e.g. "What I'm thinking now is....")

31. **Explains rationale** for questions or parts of physical examination that could appear to be non-sequiturs

32. During **physical examination**, explains process, asks permission

# EXPLANATION AND PLANNING

### Providing the correct amount and type of information

Aims:    to give comprehensive and appropriate information
to assess each individual patient's information needs
to neither restrict or overload

33. **Chunks and checks:** gives information in assimilative chunks, checks for understanding, uses patient's response as a guide to how to proceed

34. **Assesses patient's starting point:** asks for patient's prior knowledge early on when giving information, discovers extent of patient's wish for information

35. **Asks patients what other information would be helpful**
e.g. aetiology, prognosis

36. **Gives explanation at appropriate times:** avoids giving advice, information, or reassurance prematurely

## Aiding accurate recall and understanding

Aims:    to make information easier for the patient to remember and understand

37. **Organizes explanation:** divides into discrete sections, develops a logical sequence

38. **Uses explicit categorization or signposting** (e.g. "There are three important things that I would like to discuss. 1st..." "Now, shall we move on to...")

39. **Uses repetition and summarizing** to reinforce information

40. **Uses** concise, **easily understood language,** avoids or explains jargon

41. **Uses visual methods of conveying information:** diagrams, models, written information, and instructions

42. **Checks patient's understanding** of information given (or plans made): *e.g.* by asking patient to restate in own words; clarifies as necessary

## Achieving a shared understanding: incorporating the patient's perspective

Aims:    to provide explanations and plans that relate to the patient's perspective to discover the patient's thoughts and feelings about information given

to encourage an interaction rather than one-way transmission

43. **Relates explanations to patient's perspective:** to previously elicited ideas, concerns, and expectations

44. **Provides opportunities and encourages patient to contribute:** to ask questions, seek clarification, or express doubts; responds appropriately

45. **Picks up and responds to verbal and nonverbal cues** e.g. patient's need to contribute information or ask questions, information overload, distress

46. **Elicits patient's beliefs, reactions and feelings** re information given, terms used; acknowledges and addresses where necessary

## Planning: shared decision-making

Aims:    to allow patients to understand the decision-making process

to involve patients in decision-making to the level they wish

to increase patients' commitment to plans made

47. **Shares own thinking as appropriate:** ideas, thought processes, and dilemmas

48. Involves patient:

- offers suggestions and choices rather than directives
- encourages patient to contribute their own ideas, suggestions

49. Explores management options

50. Ascertains level of involvement patient wishes in making the decision at hand

51. Negotiates a mutually acceptable plan

- signposts own position of equipoise or preference regarding available options
- determines patient's preferences

52. Checks with patient if accepts plans, if concerns have been addressed

# CLOSING THE SESSION

## Forward planning

53. **Contracts** with patient re next steps for patient and physician

54. **Safety nets,** explaining possible unexpected outcomes, what to do if plan is not working, when and how to seek help

## Ensuring appropriate point of closure

55. **Summarizes** session briefly and clarifies plan of care

56. **Final check** that patient agrees and is comfortable with plan and asks if any corrections, questions or other issues

**References:**
Kurtz SM, Silverman JD, Draper J (1998) Teaching and Learning Communication Skills in Medicine. Radcliffe Medical Press (Oxford)
Silverman JD, Kurtz SM, Draper J (1998) Skills for Communicating with Patients. Radcliffe Medical Press (Oxford)

# The Calgary-Cambridge Observation Guide (advanced model)

**Providing Structure**

- Making organisation overt
- Attending to flow

---

**Initiating the Session**

- Preparation
- Establishing initial rapport
- Identifying the reason(s) for the consultation

**Gathering Information**

- Exploration of the patient's problems to discover the:
  - ❏ Biomedical perspective    ❏ The patient's perspective
    - ❏ Background information - context

**Physical Examination**

**Explanation and Planning**

- Providing the correct amount and type of information
- Aiding accurate recall and understanding
- Achieving a shared understanding: incorporating the patient's illness framework
- Planning: shared decision making

**Closing the Session**

- Ensuring appropriate point of closure
- Forward planning

---

**Building the Relationship**

- Using appropriate non-verbal behavior
- Developing rapport
- Involving the patient

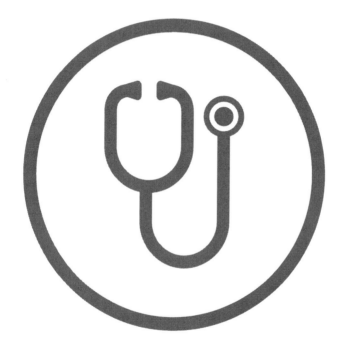

# Comskil Model for Evaluating Communication Skills Training

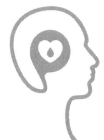

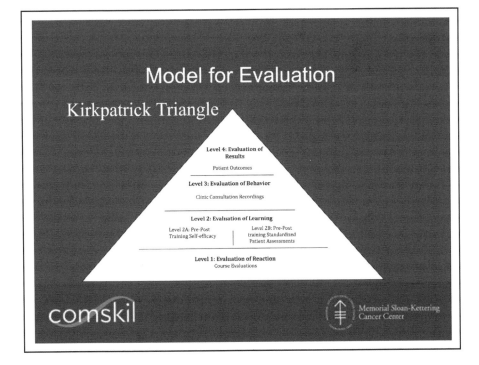

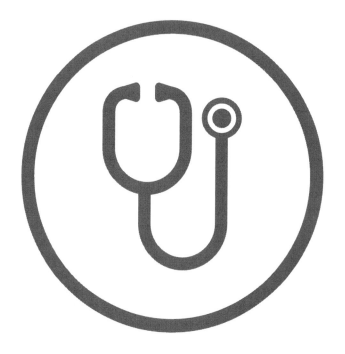

# Dealing with Anger in a Palliative Care Setting

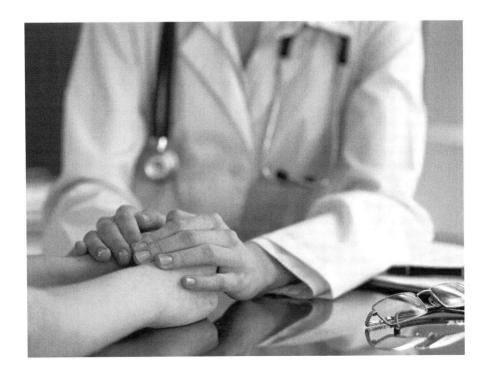

Figure 4: Some practical tips in handling anger emotion

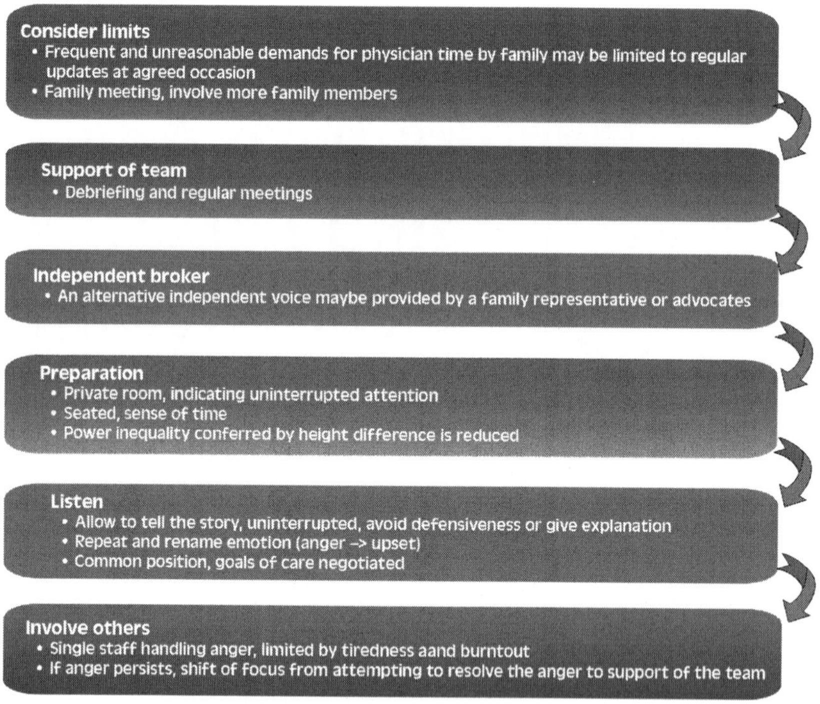

**Consider limits**
- Frequent and unreasonable demands for physician time by family may be limited to regular updates at agreed occasion
- Family meeting, involve more family members

**Support of team**
- Debriefing and regular meetings

**Independent broker**
- An alternative independent voice maybe provided by a family representative or advocates

**Preparation**
- Private room, indicating uninterrupted attention
- Seated, sense of time
- Power inequality conferred by height difference is reduced

**Listen**
- Allow to tell the story, uninterrupted, avoid defensiveness or give explanation
- Repeat and rename emotion (anger –> upset)
- Common position, goals of care negotiated

**Involve others**
- Single staff handling anger, limited by tiredness aand burntout
- If anger persists, shift of focus from attempting to resolve the anger to support of the team

Dealing with Anger in Palliative Care Setting

HKSPM Newsletter 2009 Sep Issue 2 P39

# The Palliative Performance Scale for Estimating Prognosis

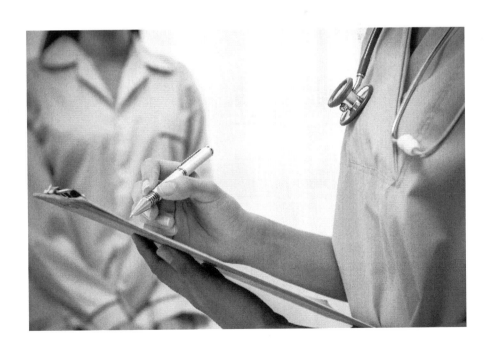

| % | Ambulation | Activity and Evidence of Disease | Self-Care | Intake | Level of Consciousness |
|---|---|---|---|---|---|
| 100 | Full | Normal Activity No Evidence of Disease | Full | Normal | Full |
| 90 | Full | Normal Activity Some Evidence of Disease | Full | Normal | Full |
| 80 | Full | Normal Activity with Effort Some Evidence of Disease | Full | Normal or Reduced | Full |
| 70 | Reduced | Unable to do Normal Job / Work Some Evidence of Disease | Full | Normal or Reduced | Full |
| 60 | Reduced | Unable to do Hobby / House Work Significant Disease | Occasional Assistance Necessary | Normal or Reduced | Full or Confusion |
| 50 | Mainly Sit/Lie | Unable to Do Any Work Extensive Disease | Considerable Assistance Required | Normal or Reduced | Full or Confusion |
| 40 | Mainly in Bed | As Above | Mainly Assistance | Normal or Reduced | Full or Drowsy or Confusion |
| 30 | Totally Bed Bound | As Above | Total Care | Reduced | Full or Drowsy or Confusion |
| 20 | As Above | As Above | Total Care | Minimal Sips | Full or Drowsy or Confusion |
| 10 | As Above | As Above | Total Care | Mouth Care Only | Drowsy or Coma |
| 0 | Death | -- | -- | -- | -- |

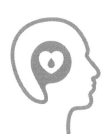

# Sample Patient History

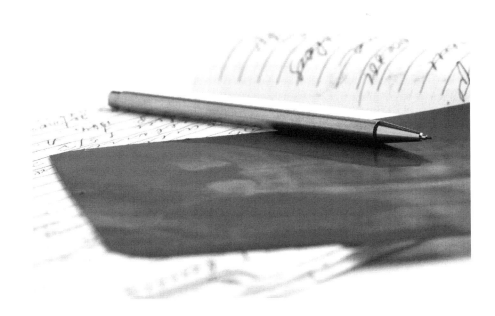

Recording the medical interview

### Patient history

Mrs G. W. 76-year-old female
Date of birth: 11/1/36 Retired shop assistant

Date: 1/6/07

**Patient's problems:**
(1) Constipation
(2) Stomach pain

**History of patient's problems:**
(1) Constipation: Started on 7/4/07. Normally bowels open once a day, but didn't go for 6 days. Subsequently has been going once every 2–4 days.
(2) Stomach pain: Pain started at the same time. Site of pain is in the left iliac fossa. Patient thought it was due to 'straining'. Episodes of pain are of sudden onset and are a 'sagging dull ache'. They last 1 hour and occur anything between 2–3 times a day to once every 3 days. There are no alleviating or exacerbating factors. Pain unrelated to eating or defecation and there are no preceding events. Pain appears not to fluctuate.
 Patient went to visit GP after 6 days constipation. GP felt a mass on abdominal palpatation which on bimanual examination was thought to be of ovarian origin. Patient referred to the gynaecological outpatient department.
 Patient does not understand why GP has referred her to hospital. Hopes the hospital can just prescribe a laxative and discharge her. Her children have arranged a holiday for her and her husband in one month's time and she does not want to miss it.

**Social history:**
Retired at age of 60 as shop assistant. Married. Husband is a retired bus driver. Alive and well. Live together in own terraced house. Self-sufficient. No pets.

**Smoking:**
Ex-smoker, 4–5 a day for 5 years as a teenager.

**Alcohol:**
Only on Christmas Day and birthdays.

**Past obstetric history:**
Menarche – 12  Menopause – 50  Gravidity 3  Parity 3

(1) Female 41  Spontaneous vaginal delivery full term (7 lb)
(2) Female 38  Spontaneous vaginal delivery full term (8 lb 4 oz)
(3) Female 35  Spontaneous vaginal delivery 39 weeks (6 lb 8 oz)

**Past medical history:**
Hypertension for last 6 years treated by GP with atenolol. No previous operations.

**Drug history:** Atenolol

**Allergies:** None known

**Travel abroad:** Never

### Family history

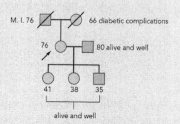

No family history of TB.

**Systems review**

**General:**
No weight change, appetite normal, no fevers, night sweats, fatigue or itch.

**Cardiovascular system:**
No chest pain, palpitations, exertional dyspnoea, paroxysmal nocturnal dyspnoea, orthopnoea or ankle oedema.

**Respiratory system:**
No cough, wheeze, sputum or haemoptysis.

**Gastrointestinal system:**
No abdominal swelling noticed by patient, no nausea or vomiting, no haematemesis. Bowels open once every 2–3 days. Stool normally formed. No blood or slime. No melaena.

**Genitourinary system:**
No dysuria, haematuria. Frequency: D 2–3, N1. No vaginal discharge. Not sexually active.

**Nervous system:**
No fits, faints or funny turns. No headache, paraesthesiae, weakness or poor balance.

**Musculoskeletal system:**
No pain or swelling of joints. Slight stiffness in morning.

**Summary:**
A 76-year-old hypertensive woman, referred to gynaecological outpatients with a short history of constipation and stomach pain. She has no other previous medical history.

**Fig. 1.5** A specimen case history taken from a student's notes. Note the brief summary at the end, the writing of which gives useful practice in the art of condensing a substantial volume of information.

# Robert Buckman's Translated "Medspeak"

| Negative | Doesn't show anything wrong |
|---|---|
| Progression | Getting worse |
| Morphologically | Under the microscope |
| Metastatic screen | Tests done to see if there has been any spread |
| Performance | How much you can do |
| Equivocal | Can't be certain what it means |
| Lung Consolidation | Pneumonia |
| Compliance | Get through the treatment |

| | |
|---|---|
| **Upper respiratory tract infection** | Cold |
| **Ecchymosis** | Bruise |
| **Postural drop** | Blood pressure goes down when you stand up |
| **Imaging** | X-ray or CT scan |
| **Partial remission** | Getting smaller |
| **Undifferentiated** | More aggressive than the average |
| **Fibrosis** | Scar tissue |
| **Neutropenia** | Low white cell count |
| **Nephropathy** | Affecting the kideys |
| **Lesion** | Something wrong |
| **Titrating** | Adjusting the dose |
| **Purpura** | Pinpoints of bleeding |
| **Vasovaginal** | Usual type of faint |
| **The bone scan is negative** | The bone scan doesn't show anything wrong |
| **There is renal dysfunction** | Your kidneys are not working normally |
| **The metastatic potential** | The chance of it spreading |

| | |
|---|---|
| **Hypertension** | High blood pressure |
| **Hematuria** | Blood in your urine |
| **Ascites** | Fluid in your abdomen |
| **There are multiple opacities on the CT** | There are a lot of shadows on the CT |
| **Equivocal significance** | We don't know if it matters or not |
| **Ischemic heart disease** | Problems with your coronary arteries |
| **It is lymph node positive** | It has spread to the lymph nodes |
| **Blast Cells** | Leukemia |
| **Demyelination** | Multiple Sclerosis |
| **Abnormal Growth** | Tumor |
| **Space occupying lesion** | Tumor |
| **The prognosis is guarded** | The situation is serious |

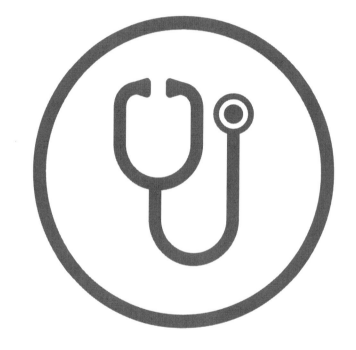

# A Chart of Applicable Laws and Regulations for Surrogate Decision Makers

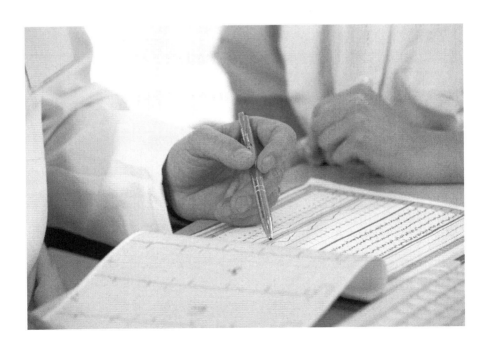

| Follow the rules in the first row that applies: | Decisions in Hospitals (excluding MH unit) and Nursing Homes | |
|---|---|---|
| | **A**<br>Consent to Treatment | **B**<br>Decision to withdraw or withhold life-sustaining treatment (including entering a DNR Order) |
| 1 | Patient, previously when capable, left prior written or oral directions | Follow patient's prior oral or written directions | Follow:<br>(i) patient's prior written directions, or<br>(ii) patient's prior oral directions if made during hospitalization before two witnesses |
| 2 | Patient, previously when capable, appointed health care agent* | Health care agent decides per PHL 29-C | Health care agent decides per PHL 29-C |
| 3 | Patient has court-appointed guardian per MHL Art 81 with health care decision-making authority.* | Guardian with health care decision-making authority decides per the FHCDA[20] | Guardian with health care decision-making authority decides per the FHCDA[21] |
| 4 | Patient resides in community (including an OMH-licensed residence) and has family or close friend* | Surrogate decides per FHCDA[22] | Surrogate decides per FHCDA[23] |
| 5 | Patient resides in community (including and OMH-licensed residence) but has no family or close friend* | (i) Surrogate Decision Making Committee (SDMC) decides per MHL Art 80 if the patient is eligible [24]<br>(ii) Otherwise, attending physician decides per FHCDA.[25] | Attending physician or court decides, per FHCDA[26] |
| 6 | Patient brought to hospital or NH from OMH-licensed or operated psych hospital or unit. Patient has family or close friend.* | (i) If patient was discharged from the OMH-licensed or operated psych hospital or unit, then surrogate decides per FHCDA.[27]<br>(ii) If patient was not discharged, then spouse, parent or adult child decides per 14 NYCRR §27.9. | (i) For DNR, surrogate decides per PHL Art 29-B<br>(ii) For other decisions, surrogate decides per FHCDA[28] |
| 7 | Patient brought to hospital or NH from OMH-licensed or operated psych hospital or unit. Patient has no family or close friend* | Decision by either<br>(i) SDMC per MHL Art 80.<br>(ii) Court per §27.9[29] | (i) For DNR, attending phys'n decides per PHL Art. 29-B<br>(ii) For other decisions, attending physician or court decides, per FHCDA.[30] |

\* Applies only if no row above it applies.

| Follow the rules in the first row that applies: | Decisions in Hospitals and Nursing Homes | |
|---|---|---|
| | **A**<br>Consent to treatment | **B**<br>Decision to withdraw or withhold life-sustaining treatment (including entering a DNR Order) |
| 1 | Patient, previously when capable, left prior written or oral directions | Follow patient's prior oral or written directions[4] | Follow:<br>(i) patient's prior written directions, or<br>(ii) patient's prior oral directions if made during hospitalization before two witnesses[5] |
| 2 | Patient, previously when capable, appointed health care agent* | Health care agent decides per PHL 29-C[6] | Health care agent decides per PHL 29-C[7] |
| 3 | Patient has a court-appointed guardian per SCPA Art. 17-A* | Guardian decides per SCPA §1750-b[8] | Guardian decides per SCPA §1750-b[9] |
| 4 | Patient resides in community (and not an OPWDD licensed residence) and has involved family* | Surrogate decides per FHCDA[10] | Involved family member decides per SCPA §1750-b.[11]<br>The prioritized list of qualified family member is set forth in 14 NYCRR §633.10(a)(7)(iv)(c). Note – A domestic partner or close friend would not qualify.[12] |
| 5 | Patient resides in community (and not an OPWDD licensed residence) but has no involved family* | Surrogate Decision Making Committee (SDMC) decides per MHL Art. 80. [13] | SDMC decides per SCPA §1750-b[14] |
| 6 | Patient resides in OPWDD-licensed or operated facility, is temporarily in a hospital or NH, and has involved family* | Involved family member decides per 14 NYCRR §633.11[15] | Involved family member decides per SCPA §1750-b.<br>The prioritized list of qualified family member is set forth in 14 NYCRR §633.10(a)(7)(iv)(c).[16] Note – A domestic partner or close friend would not qualify. |
| 7 | Patient resides in OPWDD-licensed or operated facility, is temporarily in the hospital or NH, but has no involved family* | SDMC decides per 14 NYCRR §633.11 | SDMC decides per SCPA §1750-b.[17] |

\* Applies only if no row above it applies.

# Supportive & Palliative Care Indicator Tool

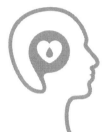

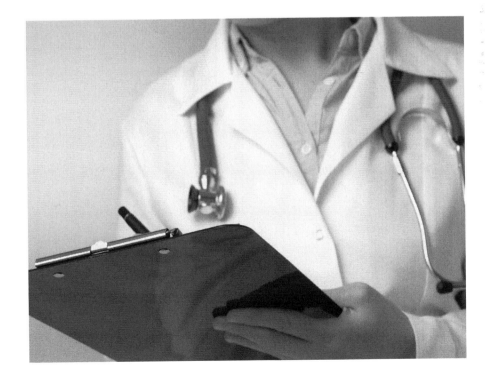

# Identifying patients for supportive and palliative care

Lothian

## Supportive & Palliative Care Indicators Tool

### 1. Ask

Would it be a surprise if this patient died in the next 6-12 months?     **No**

### 2. Look for two or more general clinical indicators

Performance status poor (limited self care; in bed or chair over 50% of the day) or deteriorating.

Progressive weight loss (>10%) over the past 6 months.

Two or more unplanned admissions in the past 6 months.

A new diagnosis of a progressive, life limiting illness.

Two or more advanced or complex conditions (multi-morbidity).

Patient is in a nursing care home or NHS continuing care unit; or needs more care at home.

### 3. Now look for two or more disease related indicators

| Heart disease | Respiratory disease | Cancer |
|---|---|---|
| NYHA Class III/IV heart failure, severe valve disease or extensive coronary artery disease. | Severe airways obstruction (FEV1 < 30%) or restrictive deficit (vital capacity < 60%, transfer factor < 40%). | Performance status deteriorating due to metastatic cancer and/ or co-morbidities. |
| Breathless or chest pain at rest or on minimal exertion. | Meets criteria for long term oxygen therapy (PaO2 < 7.3 kPa). | Persistent symptoms despite optimal palliative oncology treatment or too frail for oncology treatment. |
| Persistent symptoms despite optimal tolerated therapy. | Breathless at rest or on minimal exertion between exacerbations. | **Neurological disease** |
| Systolic blood pressure < 100mmHg and /or pulse > 100. | Persistent severe symptoms despite optimal tolerated therapy. | Progressive deterioration in physical and/or cognitive function despite optimal therapy. |
| Renal impairment (eGFR < 30 ml/min). | Symptomatic right heart failure. | Symptoms which are complex and difficult to control. |
| Cardiac cachexia. | Low body mass index (< 21). | Speech problems with increasing difficulty communicating and/or progressive dysphagia. |
| Two or more acute episodes needing intravenous therapy in past 6 months. | More emergency admissions (> 3) for infective exacerbations or respiratory failure in past year. | Recurrent aspiration pneumonia; breathless or respiratory failure. |
| **Kidney disease** | **Liver disease** | **Dementia** |
| Stage 4 or 5 chronic kidney disease (eGFR < 30ml/min). | Advanced cirrhosis with one or more complications: | Unable to dress, walk or eat without assistance; unable to communicate meaningfully. |
| Conservative kidney management due to multi-morbidity. | • intractable ascites | |
| Deteriorating on renal replacement therapy with persistent symptoms and/or increasing dependency. | • hepatic encephalopathy<br>• hepatorenal syndrome<br>• bacterial peritonitis<br>• recurrent variceal bleeds | Worsening eating problems (dysphagia or dementia related) - now needing pureed/ soft diet or supplements. |
| Not starting dialysis following failure of a renal transplant. | Serum albumin < 25g/l and prothrombin time raised or INR prolonged (INR > 2). | Recurrent febrile episodes or infections; aspiration pneumonia. |
| New life limiting condition or kidney failure as a complication of another condition or treatment. | Hepatocellular carcinoma. | Urinary and faecal incontinence. |
| | Not fit for liver transplant. | |

### 4. Assess patient & family for supportive & palliative care needs. Review treatment/ medication. Plan care. Consider patient for general practice palliative care register.

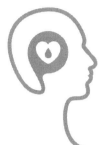

# Glossary

**Adaptive behavior.** Any behavior that enables an individual to change their disruptive behavior

**Advanced directive.** A legal document (as a living will) signed by a competent person to provide guidance for medical and health care decisions

**Amplification.** Strategy for discussing enrollment of clinical trials whereby the physician gives the patient a chance to react to the standard treatment options

just before for introducing an alternative option

**Anesthesiology.** Branch of medical science dealing with anesthesia and anesthetics

**Anticipatory grief.** A stage of mourning that occurs when a patient or family is expecting a death. Symptoms include depression, extreme concern for the dying person, preparing for the death, and adjusting to changes caused by the death

**Autonomy.** The quality or state of being self-governing

**Autosomal recessive disorder.** A disease caused by the presence of two recessive mutant genes on an autosome

**Beneficence.** Any medical action that serves the best interests of patients and promotes well-being

**Buried question.** A question, issue or concern hidden within a statement made by the patient regarding his or her medical condition

**Cardiovascular system.** An organ system that encompasses the heart and blood vessels of the body (also known as the circulatory system)

**Casuistry.** A decision-making method used in biomedical ethics whereby the physician relies on previous experience with similar cases

**Chaplain.** A member of the clergy who provides for the spiritual needs of patients and families

**Checking for understanding.** The act of asking the patient if he or she understands what the physician as just explained so as to ensure the information has been digested

**Chronic illness.** A health condition or disease that is persistent or lasting in its effects

**Chunking.** The act of breaking up information into smaller parts to increase comprehension

**Circular question.** A question designed to enable a patient or family member to see an alternative perspective; the act of asking someone to comment on the statements of another

**Clinical agenda.** The medical goals of care outlined by the physician

**Clinical relationship.** The medical relationship between the physician and the patient

**Clinical interview.** An interview conducted by a physician regarding a patient's medical status, agenda, or plan

**Clinical trial.** Tests in **medical research** and **drug development** that generate safety and **efficacy** for future health interventions

**Coercion.** The act of forcing a patient to make a desired medical decision through manipulation or some other pressure

**Cognitive appraisals.** A hypothesis or personal interpretation formed about the patient's needs based on a hinted or explicit narrative

**Consultation.** Deliberation by two or more physicians about diagnosis or treatment in a particular case

**Cognitive function.** Introverted or extroverted mental functions of thinking, feeling, sensing and intuition

**Collective equipoise.** The right of a medical team to make a choice for the patient when the patient demonstrates indifference between two choices

**Communication goals.** The desired outcome of a consultation

a physician wishes to achieve through communication

**Collusion.** A secretive agreement made between a physician and a patient or family member

**Complementary and alternative medicine.** Any medical practice or product not considered standard care

**CONES protocol.** An acronym designed as a strategy to disclose medical errors to patients

**Contextual meaning.** Meaning derived from any scenario defined and understood by the context of its events

**Counter-transference.** A physician's emotional or psychological entanglement with a patient created out the physician's own unresolved conflicts

**Curative care.** Any medical agenda with the intended goal of curing the patient

**Decision aid.** Any audio or visual tool used to facilitate patient decision-making

**Declaration.** Strategy for discussing enrollment of clinical trials whereby the physician tells the patient which treatment he or she feels is the best among the ones presented

**Defense mechanism.** A psychological tactic developed by the ego to protect itself against anxiety

**Diagnosis.** The act or process of identifying or determining the nature and cause of a disease or injury

**Dialysis.** The process of cleansing the blood by passing it through a special machine

**Disclosure.** A physician's act of revealing medical related information

**Displacement behavior.** The redirection of an emotion or impulse from its original object (as an idea or person) to something more acceptable

**DNR order.** Advanced directive acronym for "do not resuscitate"

**DSM-IV.** Acronym for the fourth edition of the Diagnostic and Statistical Manual of Mental Disorders, a comprehensive classification of officially recognized psychiatric disorders

**Dyadic convergence.** The convergence of two perspectives, ideas, or opinions

**Dyspnea.** A condition of difficult or labored breathing indicating a sign of serious disease of the airway, lungs, or heart

**Efficacy.** A treatment that has the power to produce an effect

**Empathy.** The capacity to recognize and relate to an emotional experience

**Emotional data.** Information about the patient provided to the physician via the patient's emotional response

**Emotional temperature.** The intensity of emotion demonstrated by the patient

**Empathic statement.** A listening technique framed

as an emotional restatement that verbally names an emotion expressed by the patient

**Enunciation.** Strategy for discussing enrollment of clinical trials whereby the physician elicits the patient's preference among treatment options

**Error disclosure.** The act of revealing a medical error to the patient

**Existential anxiety.** A sense of worry, dread or panic that may arise from the contemplation of life's biggest questions

**Gastrointestinal system.** The biological system that makes food absorbable into the body

**Genitourinary system.** The body's reproductive organs and the urinary system

**Grief cycle.** The range of emotions experienced by a patient diagnosed with a serious illness

**HARD strategy.** Acronym for the four-step strategy to dealing

with conflict escalation between patients, physicians, and/or family members

**Hippocratic oath.** An oath taken by physicians upon entering the practice of medicine to uphold the established duties and obligations of medicine

**Hospice care.** A form of palliative care offered in a home setting

**Ideation.** The act of forming or entertaining ideas

**Independent broker.** A third party brought in to resolve a difference of ideas and opinions between two other parties

**Individual equipoise.** A state of equilibrium whereby a patient expresses no partiality between two choices

**Informed consent.** A process of communication between a patient and physician resulting in the patient's authorization or agreement to undergo a specific medical intervention

**Illness trajectory.** The predicted or documented path of an illness

**Interquartile range.** A measure of **statistical range**, being equal to the difference between the upper and lower **quartiles**

**Intervention intensity.** The degree to which a physician intervenes in the patient's decision-making process

**Karnofsky Performance Scale.** An index that classifies patients according to their functional impairment

**Kubler-Ross model.** Theoretical model of the grief cycle

**Maladaptive behavior.** Any patient behavior considered detrimental to the patient's medical situation and/or goals of care

**Malpractice.** Failure of a physician to render proper services through reprehensible ignorance or negligence or through criminal intent, especially when injury or personal loss follows

**Management plan.** The physician's plan to treat, cure, or manage an illness

**Medical history.** A collection of information obtained from the patient and from other sources concerning the patient's physical status as well as his or her psychological, social, and sexual function

**Median rates.** A numerical value separating the higher half of a data sample

**Med-speak.** Technical jargon and abbreviations used among health care professionals to communicate

**Metastatic.** The transference of disease-producing organisms to other parts of the body by way of the blood cells, lymphatic vessels, or membranous surfaces

**Musculoskeletal system.** The biological system of muscles, tendons, ligaments, bones, joints, and tissues that move the body

**Nervous system.** The system of cells, tissues, and organs that regulates the body's responses to internal and external stimuli

**Neurology.** The medical specialty concerned with the diagnosis and treatment of nervous system disorders

**Neurosurgery.** Surgery of the brain or other nerve tissue

**Next of kin.** A patient's closest living blood relative or relatives

**Non-maleficence.** The ethical principle of doing no harm

**Non-small cell lung cancer.** Cancer that accounts for nearly nine out of every ten cases and usually grows at a slower rate than small cell lung cancer

**Nonverbal cues.** Perceptual information communicated in through body language

**NURSE protocol.** Acronym for a protocol that attempts to identify a patient's emotion

**Oncology.** Branch of medical science that studies cancer

**Open question.** A question that requires a developed answer beyond yes or no

**Osteochondroses.** A disease of bone and cartilage in children

**Outpatient.** A patient who receives treatment at a hospital, but is not hospitalized

**Over-dependency.** The state of becoming too reliant on someone or something for aid

**Palliative care.** A method of administering comfort care and pain management offered by hospitals

**Paternalistic approach.** The medical approach of making all the patient's decisions and providing information as seen fit

**Patient agenda.** The patient's concerns and desired outcome for their health care

**Patient barriers.** Anything that prevents the patient from taking an action or reaching compliance

**Patient-centered.** The medical approach of considering the patient's values in the goals of care

**Patient narrative.** The patient's story of the illness

**Patient values.** Qualities the patient feels are important in their life as it relates to medical care

**Phase 1 clinical trial.** The research stage at which researchers test a new drug on a small group of people for the first time to evaluate its safety, determine a safe dosage range, and identify side effects

**Phase 2 clinical trial.** The research stage at which a new drug or treatment is given to a larger group of people to see if it is effective and to further evaluate its safety

**Phase 3 clinical trial.** The research stage at which a new drug or treatment given to large groups of people to confirm its effectiveness and safety

**Physician barriers.** Anything that prevents the physician from taking an action or reaching compliance

**Physician agenda.** The physician's concerns and desired outcome for the patient's health care

**Primary care physician.** A physician chosen by an individual to serve as his or her health care professional

**Process tasks.** Dialogues and nonverbal behaviors that create an environment for effective communication

**Prognosis.** The forecast of the probable outcome or course of a disease, including the patient's chance of recovery

**Prognostic error.** A forecasting error regarding the course of a disease or the patient's chance of recovery

**Prognostic interview.** A meeting arranged by the physician with the patient and/or family to talk about the patient's medical prognosis

**Psychohistory.** The study of the events in an individual's life that determine psychological motivations

**Psychosocial.** A person's psychological development in relation to the social environment

**Quality of life.** The general well-being of a patient in normal society

**Reflexive question.** A question that elicits brainstorming of possibilities or future outcomes

**Relational conflict.** A conflict between two relatives over the goals of patient care

**Remission.** The period in the course of a disease when symptoms become less severe

**Risk factor.** Something that increases risk or susceptibility

**Roter interactional analysis scheme.** A method for coding medical dialogue

**Shielding.** The act of withholding information from a patient or relative to ease the burden of suffering

**Side effects.** An effect of treatment that is secondary to the effect intended

**Staging.** The process of determining the extent to which a cancer has developed through spreading

**Standard treatment.** Treatment normally provided to people with a given condition

**Small lung cancer.** Cancer that resembles "oats" under a microscope, begins in the lung tissue, and spreads quickly

**Somatic.** Relating to the body

**SPIKES protocol.** Acronym for the protocol designed to disclose medical errors

**Spirituality.** A term for the state of being that transcends beyond the biological body

**Strategic question.** A question designed to guide families toward decisions without seeming intrusive

**Surrogate decision maker.** A relative or friend appointed to act as the decision maker on behalf of a mentally incapable patient

**Survival rates.** The percentage of people with a disease who remain alive for a given period of time after diagnosis

**Survivorship.** The state of being a survivor of a disease

**Sympathy.** The state of having an understanding of another person's situation

**Symptom.** Any expected change in the body that accompanies a disease

**Symptomatic relief.** The alleviation of expected changes in the body caused by a disease

**Symptom management.** Care given to improve the quality of life of patients who experience biological changes from a serious or life-threatening disease

**System failure analysis.** An analysis conducted by a medical team to determine the cause of a systemic breakdown in medical care in order to prevent it from happening again

**Terminal phase.** The last phase of a disease; the dying phase

**Theoretical model.** A model introduced in a non-specific way as a guideline or concept

**Therapy.** A treatment intended to prevent a medical condition from occurring

**Transition point.** The point at which a **boundary layer** changes

**Treatment regimen.** A regulated plan designed to yield a positive result

**Triadic convergence.** The convergence of at least three perspectives, ideas, or opinions

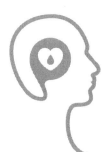

# Bibliography

Aafp.org. "How to Manage Difficult Patient Encounters." **www.aafp.org/fpm/2007/0600/p30.html**, Family Practice Management, 2007 Vol. 14 No. 6.

Aans.org. "Informed Consent." **www.aans.org/en/Education%20and% 20Meetings/CME/~/media/Files/Education%20and%20Meetingf/ Ethics%20Module/13InformedConsentModuleWTC35.ashx**, 2013.

Acponline.org. "Beyond Symptom Management." **www.acponline. org/ebizatpro/images/productimages/books/sample%20chapters/ Physicians%20Guide%20to%20End%20Of%20Life_Ch04.pdf**, 2001.

Annals.org. "Risk Management: Extreme Honesty May Be the Best Policy." **http://annals.org/article.aspx?articleid=713181**, 1999, Vol. 131. No. 12.

Back, Anthony; Arnold, Robert; Tulsky, James. *Mastering Communication with Seriously Ill Patients.* The Cambridge University Press, 2009.

Bensing, Jozien; Jan Kerssens; and Marja van der Pasch. Patient-Directed Gaze as a Tool for Discovering and Handling Psychosocial Problems in General Practice," *Journal of Nonverbal Behavior 19(4), Winter 1995.*

Berry J.W.; U. Kim, T.; Minde, et al. *Comparative studies of acculturative stress.* Internal Migraine Review, 1987.

Bmj.com. "Extent and Determinants of Error in Doctors' Prognoses in Terminally Ill Patients: Prospective Cohort Study." **www.bmj.com/content/320/7233/469**, 2000.

Buckman, Robert, How to Break Bad News: A guide for health care professionals. The John Hopkins University Press, 1992.

Buckman, Robert, *Difficult Conversations in Medicine.* The John Hopkins University Press, 2010.

Butow P.N.; R.F. Brown; S. Cogar, et al. *Oncologists reactions to cancer patients verbal cues.* Psycho-Oncology, 2002.

Canceremotionalwellbeing.com. Interview With Breast Surgeon Dr. Deanna Attai, Part 1. **www.canceremotionalwellbeing.com/2012/06/interview-with-breast-surgeon-dr-deanna-attai-part-1/**, 2012.

Caregiver.org. "End-of-Life Decision Making." **www.caregiver.org/caregiver/jsp/content_node.jsp?nodeid=401**, 2013.

Changingminds.org. *"On Death and Dying,"* Macmillan: New York, 1969. **http://changingminds.org/disciplines/change_management/kubler_ross/kubler_ross.htm**, 2013

Christianhealth.com. "Religion, Spirituality, and Medicine: A Rebuttal To Skeptics." **http://christianhealth.com/health/health05.html**, International Journal of Psychiatry in Medicine Vol. 29 No. 2, 1999.

Cohen-Cole, Steven. The Medical Interview: The Three-Function Approach. Mosby-Year, 1991.

Conflictandhealth.com. "Ethics of Conducting Research in Conflict Settings." **www.conflictandhealth.com/content/3/1/7**, 2009.

Dartmouth-hitchcock.org. "Developing Ethical Strategies to Assist Oncologists in Seeking Informed Consent to Cancer Clinical Trials." **www.dartmouth-hitchcock.org/dhmc-internet-upload/ file_collection/Brown%20RF.pdf**, Social Science & Medicine Vol. 58, 379–390, 2004.

Doctorquality.com. "Systems Approach to Improving Error Reporting." **www.doctorquality.com/www/docs/joshi.pdf**, 2013.

Erj.ersjournals.com. Palliative and end-of-life care for patients with severe COPD. **http://erj.ersjournals.com/content/32/3/796.full**, 2013.

Fmshk.org, "Dealing with Anger in a Palliative Care Setting." **www.fmshk.org/database/articles/hkspmnewslettersep09p3639 dealingwithangerinpalliativecare.pdf**, 2009.

Healthcarecommunication.org. "Agenda Setting in the Medical Interview." **www.healthcarecommunication.org/pro/hcrps/ PSArticle2.pdf**, 2001.

Healthteamworks-media.precis5.com. "Discrepant Perceptions About End-of-Life Communication: A Systematic Review." **http://health teamworks-media.precis5.com/8248a99e81e752cb9b41da3fc43fbe7f**, Journal of Pain and Symptom Management Vol. 34 No. 2, August 2007.

Jeramyt.org. "Casuistry — A Summary." www.jeramyt.org/papers/casuistry.html, 2003.

Jco.ascopubs.org, "Cancer Patient Preferences for Communication of Prognosis in the Metastatic Setting." http://jco.ascopubs.org/content/22/9/1721.full.pdf, 2004.

Jco.ascopubs.org. "Discussing Prognosis: 'How Much Do You Want to Know?' Talking to Patients Who Are Prepared for Explicit Information." http://jco.ascopubs.org/content/24/25/4209.long, 2006.

Jco.ascopubs.org. "Necessary Collusion: Prognostic Communication with Advanced Cancer Patients." http://jco.ascopubs.org/content/23/13/3146.full.pdf, 2005.

Journal.nzma.org.nz, "The immediate and Long-Term Impact on New Zealand Doctors who Receive Patient Complaints." http://journal.nzma.org.nz/journal/117-1198/972/. Journal of the New Zealand Medical Association, 23-July-2004, Vol 117 No 1198.

Kissane, David; Parry Bultz; Phylliss Butow; and Ilora Finlay. *The Handbook of Communication and Oncology in Palliative Care.* The Oxford University Press, 2010.

Lind, Stuart; Mary-Jo Del Vecchio; Steven Seidel; Thomas Csordas; and Byron Good. Telling the diagnosis of Cancer. *Journal of Clinical Oncology,* Vol 7, No 5 (May), 1989: pp 583-589. http://webcache.googleusercontent.com/search?q=cache:BSRro0LcyRYJ:jco.ascopubs.org/content/7/5/583.full.pdf+telling+the+diagnosis+of+cancer&cd=1&hl=en&ct=clnk&gl=us, 2013

Marvel, Kim; Ronald Epstein; Kristine Flowers; and Howard Beckman. Soliciting the Patient's Agenda Journal of American Medicine, Vol. 281 No. 3, 1999.

Mdm.sagepub.com. "Rethinking the Objectives of Decision Aids: A Call for Conceptual Clarity." **http://chicago.medicine.uic.edu/ UserFiles/Servers/Server_442934/File/OBGYN/Critique%20 of%20clinical%20equipoise.%20hastings.%20center%20report.pdf.** Medical Decision Making, 2007.

Medicaltextbooksrevealed.s3.amazonaws.com. "Consultation, Medical History and Record Taking." **http://medicaltextbooksrevealed. s3.amazonaws.com/files/17028-53.pdf,** 2013.

Medicaring.org. "Adapting Health Care to Serious Chronic Illness in Old Age." **http://medicaring.org/whitepaper/,** 2003.

Medscape.org. "Communicating With Cancer Patients: When the News Is Bad." **www.medscape.org/viewarticle/585837,** 2009.

Medscape.org. "A Question of Ethics: An Expert Interview With Amy Brodkey, MD." **www.medscape.com/viewarticle/713480,** 2009.

Medstation.yale.edu. "Principles and Practice of Withdrawing Life-Sustaining Treatments." **http://medstation.yale.edu/picu/files/www/ Articles/EOL/Practice_of_withdrawing.pdf.** Critical Care Clinics, Vol. 20, 2004.

Med.unc.edu. "Patient-centered clinical method." **www.med.unc.edu/epic/module7/m7a2a.htm,** 2013.

Ncbi.nlm.nih.gov. "Existential Loneliness and End-of-Life Care: A Systematic Review." **www.ncbi.nlm.nih.gov/pmc/articles/ PMC2866502/?tool=pubmed.** Theoretical Medical Bioethics, Vol. 31 No 2, 2010.

Ncbi.nlm.nih.gov. Kessels, Roy. Journal of the Royal Society of Medicine. 2003 May; 96(5): 219–222. **www.ncbi.nlm.nih.gov/pmc/articles/PMC539473/**, 2003.

Ncbi.nlm.nih.gov. Lichstein, Peter R. "Clinical Methods: The History, Physical, and Laboratory Examinations." **www.ncbi.nlm.nih.gov/books/NBK349/**, 1990.

Ncbi.nlm.nih.gov. "Preferred Roles in Treatment Decision Making Among Patients With Cancer: A Pooled Analysis of Studies Using the Control Preferences Scale." **www.ncbi.nlm.nih.gov/pmc/articles/PMC3020073/, 2010.**

Ncbi.nlm.nih.gov. "When Does Primary Care Turn into Palliative Care?" **www.ncbi.nlm.nih.gov/pmc/articles/PMC1071520/**, Western Journal of Medicine, Vol. 175 No. 3, 2001.

Nejm.org. "Managing Conflict at the End of Life." **www.nejm.org/doi/full/10.1056/NEJMp058104**, 2005.

Onlinelibrary.wiley.com "The language divide: the importance of training in the use of interpreters for outpatient practice." **http://onlinelibrary.wiley.com/doi/10.1111/j.1525-1497.2004.30268.x/full**, 2004.

Palliative.info. "Guideline for Estimating Length of Survival in Palliative Patients." **http://palliative.info/teaching_material/Prognosis.pdf,** 2013.

Palliative.info. "Health Care Professional — Educational Resources and Programs." **http://palliative.info/pages/Education.htm**, 2013.

Pediatrics.aapublications.org, "Gaps in Doctor-Patient Communication," American Academy of Pediatrics, 1968.

http://pediatrics.aappublications.org/content/42/5/855.abstract?lin kType=ABST&journalCode=pediatrics&resid=42/5/855, 2013.

Philological.net. "Interview with an Oncologist on Doctor-Patient Interactions." www.philologica.net/studia/20110121233000. htm, 2011.

PsychCentral.com, "Nonverbal Cues Influence Physician-Patient Encounters." http://psychcentral.com/news/2011/09/27/nonverbal-cues-influence-physician-patient-encounters/29807.html, 2011.

Ptjournal.com. "Reducing Medical Errors: An Organizational Approach." http://ptjournal.com/ptJournal/fulltext/28/12/ PTJ2812780.pdf, 2003.

Radiology.rsna.org. "Radiology Failure Mode and Effect Analysis: What Is It?" http://radiology.rsna.org/content/252/2/544.full, 2009.

Roter, Deborah; and Judith Hall. Doctors Talking with Patients/ Patients Talking with Doctors. Praeger House, 2006.

Skillscascade.com, *Marrying Content and Process in Clinical Method Teaching: Enhancing the Calgary–Cambridge Guides.* www. skillscascade.com/files/acmed03.pdf. Academic Medicine , Vol. 78 No. 8, August 2003.

Thefreelibrary.com. "Conflict Management, Prevention, and Resolution in Medical Settings." www.thefreelibrary.com/Conflict+management %2c+prevention%2c+and+resolution+in+medical+settings.... -a0102342542, 1999.

Thepermanentejournal.org, "Getting the Most out of the Clinical Encounter: The Four Habits Model." http://xnet.kp.org/ permanentejournal/fall99pj/habits.html, 1999.

Trialsjournal.com. "Does Clinical Equipoise Apply to Cluster Randomized Trials in Health Research?" **www.trialsjournal.com/ content/pdf/1745-6215-12-118.pdf**, Vol 12 No. 118, 2011.

Turkailehekderg.org, "The patient-centered clinical method: a family medicine perspective." **www.turkailehekderg.org/Port_Doc/ TAHD_2013/TAHD_2013002/TAHD_2013002007.pdf**, 2013

Uic.edu. "Surrogate Decision Making," **www.uic.edu/depts/mcam/ ethics/surrogate.htm**, 2013.

Utcomchatt.org. "Principles of Biomedical Ethics." **www.utcomchatt. org/docs/biomedethics.pdf**. Erlanger Medical Ethics Orientation Manual, 2000.

Ww1.cpa-apc.org. "Psychotherapeutic Interventions at the End of Life: A Focus on Meaning and Spirituality." **ww1.cpa-apc.org:8080/ publications/archives/CJP/2004/june/breitbart.pdf**. Canada Journal of Psychiatry, Vol. 49, No 6, 2004.

www2.edc.org. "Taking a Spiritual History Allows Clinicians to Understand Patients More Fully: An Interview with Dr. Christina Puchalski." **www2.edc.org/lastacts/archives/archivesNov99/ featureinn.asp**, 1999.

www.interscience.wiley.com, "The Communication Goals and Needs of Cancer Patients: A Review." **http://people.ucalgary.ca/~lcarlso/ Hack%20comm%20needs%20PON.pdf**, 2005.

www.ncbi.nlm.nih.gov. "The Effects of Cultural Differences on the Physician-Patient Relationship." **www.ncbi.nlm.nih.gov/pmc/ articles/PMC2328087/pdf/canfamphys00192-0175.pdf**. Canadian Family Physician, Vol. 32, 1986.

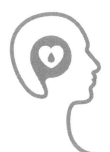

# Index

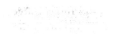

# About the Author

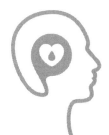

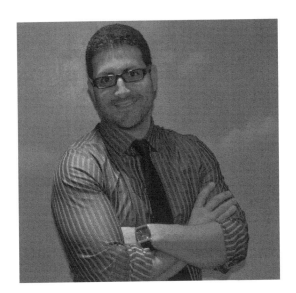

ichael J. Cavallaro was born in New Hyde Park, New York, and was educated at Villanova University. Following his years as an editor with HarperCollins Publishers, he has worked as a freelance technical writer for commercial business. This is his fourth book.

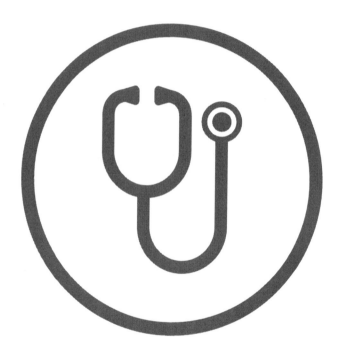